THE
FEMALE REPRODUCTIVE SYSTEM

ATLAS *of* TUMOR RADIOLOGY

PHILIP J. HODES, M.D., *Editor-in-Chief*

Sponsored by

THE AMERICAN COLLEGE OF RADIOLOGY

—*with the cooperation of:*

AMERICAN CANCER SOCIETY
AMERICAN ROENTGEN RAY SOCIETY
CANCER CONTROL PROGRAM, USPHS
EASTMAN KODAK COMPANY
JAMES PICKER FOUNDATION
RADIOLOGICAL SOCIETY OF NORTH AMERICA

THE
FEMALE
REPRODUCTIVE SYSTEM

by

G. MELVIN STEVENS, M.D., M.S. (Radiol.)

Department of Radiology, Palo Alto Clinic;
Clinical Associate Professor of Radiology,
Stanford University School of Medicine, Palo Alto, Calif.

YEAR BOOK MEDICAL PUBLISHERS · INC.
35 EAST WACKER DRIVE, CHICAGO

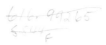

Library of Congress Catalog Card Number: 72-147397

International Standard Book Number: 0-8151-8240-9

Printed in U.S.A.

Dedicated to

RUTH, GRANT, CHARLES *and* SUSAN

Editor's Preface

In 1960, the Committee on Radiology of the National Research Council began to consider the preparation of a tumor atlas for radiology similar in concept to the Armed Forces Institute of Pathology's "Atlas of Tumor Pathology." So successfully had the latter filled a need in pathology that it seemed reasonable to establish a similar resource for radiology. Therefore a subcommittee of the Committee on Radiology was appointed to study the concept and make recommendations.

That original committee, made up of Dr. Russell H. Morgan (Chairman), Dr. Marshall H. Brucer and Dr. Eugene P. Pendergrass, reported that a need did indeed exist and recommended that something be done about it. That report was unanimously accepted by the parent committee.

Soon thereafter, there occurred a normal change of the membership of the Committee on Radiology of the Council. This was followed by a change of the "Atlas" subcommittee, which now included Dr. E. Richard King (Chairman), Dr. Leo G. Rigler and Dr. Barton R. Young. To this new subcommittee was assigned the task of finding how the "Atlas" was to be published. Numerous avenues were explored; none seemed wholly satisfactory.

With the passing of time, it became increasingly apparent that the American College of Radiology had to be brought into the picture. It had prime teaching responsibilities; it had a Commission on Education; it seemed the logical responsible agent to launch the "Atlas." Confident of the merits of this approach, the entire Committee on Radiology of the Council became involved in focusing the attention of the American College of Radiology upon the matter.* In 1964, as the result of their persuasiveness, the Board of Chancellors of the American College of Radiology named an ad hoc committee to explore and define the scholarly scope of the "Atlas" and the probable costs. In 1965, the ad hoc committee recommended that the College sponsor and publish the "Atlas." Accordingly, an Editorial Advisory Com-

---

* At that time, the Committee on Radiology included, in addition to the subcommittee, Drs. John A. Campbell, James B. Dealy, Jr., Melvin M. Figley, Hymer L. Friedell, Howard B. Latourette, Alexander Margulis, Ernest A. Mendelsohn, Charles M. Nice, Jr., and Edward W. Webster.

mittee was chosen to work within the Commission on Education with authority to select an Editor-in-Chief. At the same time, the College provided funds for starting the project and began representations for grants-in-aid without which the "Atlas" would never be published.

No history of the "Atlas of Tumor Radiology" would be complete without specific recording of the generous response of the several radiological societies, as well as the private and Federal granting institutions whose names appear on the title page and below among our acknowledgments. It was their tangible evidence of confidence in the project that provided everyone with enthusiasm and eagerness to achieve our goal.

The "Atlas of Tumor Radiology" includes all major organ systems. It is intended to be a systematic body of pictorial and written information dealing with the roentgen manifestations of tumors. No attempt has been made to provide an atlas equivalent of a medical encyclopedia. Nevertheless the "Atlas" is designed to serve as an important reference source and teaching file for all physicians, not radiologists alone.

The thirteen volumes of the "Atlas," to be completed in 1971-72, are: *The Hemopoietic and Lymphatic Systems*, by Gerald D. Dodd and Sidney Wallace; *The Bones and Joints*, by Gwilym Lodwick; *The Lower Respiratory Tract and Thoracic Contents*, by Roy R. Greening and J. Haynes Heslep; *The Gastrointestinal Tract*, by Arthur K. Finkelstein and George N. Stein; *The Upper Urinary Tract,* by John A. Evans and Morton A. Bosniak (published); *The Lower Urinary Tract,* by John A. Evans and Morton A. Bosniak; *The Breast,* by David M. Witten (published); *The Head and Neck,* by Gilbert H. Fletcher and Bao-Shan Jing (published); *The Brain and Eye*, by Ernest W. Wood, Juan M. Taveras and Michael S. Tenner; *The Female Reproductive System*, by G. Melvin Stevens (published); *The Endocrines*, by Howard L. Steinbach and Hideyo Minagi (published); *The Accessory Digestive Organs*, by Robert E. Wise; and *The Spine*, by Bernard S. Epstein.

Some overlapping of material in several volumes is inevitable, for example, tumors of the female generative system, tumors of the endocrine glands and tumors of the urinary tract. This is considered to be an asset. It assures the specialist completeness in the volume or volumes that concern him and provides added breadth and depth of knowledge for those interested in the entire series.

The broad scope of the "Atlas of Tumor Radiology" has precluded its preparation by a single or even several authors. To maintain uniformity of format, rather rigid criteria were established early. These included manner of presentation, size of illustrations, as well as style of headings, subheadings and legends. The authors were encouraged to keep the text at a minimum, freeing as much space as possible for large illustrations and meaningful legends. The "Atlas" is to be just that, an "atlas," not a series of "texts." The authors were urged, also, to keep the bibliography brief.

The selection of suitable authors for the "Atlas" was extremely difficult, and to a degree invidious. For the final choice, the Editor-in-Chief accepts full responsibility. It is but fair to record, however, that his Editorial Advisory Committee accepted his recommendations. The format of the "Atlas," too, was the choice of the Editor-in-Chief, again with the concurrence of his advisory group. Should the "Atlas of Tumor Radiology" fall short of its goals, the fault will lie with the Editor-in-Chief alone; his Editorial Advisory Committee was selfless in its dedication to the purposes of the "Atlas," rendering invaluable advice and guidance whenever asked to do so.

As medical knowledge expands, medical concepts change. In medicine, the written word considered true today may not be so tomorrow. The text of the "Atlas," considered true today, therefore may not be true tomorrow. What may not change, what may ever remain true, may be the illustrations of the "Atlas of Tumor Radiology." Their legends may change as our conceptual levels advance. But the validity of the roentgen findings there recorded should endure. Thus, if the fidelity with which the roentgenograms have been reproduced is of superior order, the illustrations in the "Atlas" should long serve as sources for reference no matter what revisions of the text become necessary with advancing medical knowledge.

ACKNOWLEDGMENTS

The American College of Radiology, its Commission on Education, the Editorial Advisory Committee, the authors and the Editor-in-Chief wish to acknowledge their grateful appreciation:

1. For the grants-in-aid so willingly and repeatedly provided by The American Cancer Society, The American Roentgen Ray Society, The Cancer Control Program, National Center for Chronic Disease Control (USPHS Grant No. 59481), The James Picker Foundation, and The Radiological Society of North America.

2. For the superb glossy print reproductions provided by the Radiography Markets Division, Eastman Kodak Company. Special mention must be made of the sustained interest of Mr. George R. Struck, its Assistant Vice-President and General Manager. We applaud particularly Mr. William S. Cornwell, Technical Associate and Editor Emeritus of Kodak's *Medical Radiography and Photography,* as well as his associates, Mr. Charles C. Heckman and Mr. Stanley J. Pietrzkowski and others in the Photo Service

Division, whose expertise provided the "Atlas" with its incomparable photographic reproductions.

3. To Year Book Medical Publishers, for their personal involvement with and judicious guidance in the many problems of publication. There were occasions when the publisher questioned the quality of certain illustrations. Almost always the judgment of the authors and the Editor-in-Chief prevailed because of the importance of the original roentgenograms and the singular fidelity of their reproduction.

4. To the Associate Editors, particularly Mrs. Anabel I. Janssen, whose talents lightened the burden of the Editor-in-Chief and helped establish the style of presentation of the material.

5. To the Staff of the American College of Radiology, especially Messrs. William C. Stronach, Otha Linton, Keith Gundlach and William Melton, for continued conceptual and administrative efforts of unusual competence.

Few American authors have had Dr. Stevens's range of experience with tumors of the female pelvis. Despite this, he chose to invite the cooperation of several foreign colleagues whose knowledge in certain regards he considered even greater than his. By so doing Dr. Stevens has again demonstrated his dedication to excellence which has been the hallmark of his professional career.

The "Atlas of Tumor Radiology" is being published in a time when massive scientific effort is taking place at an unprecedented rate and on an unprecedented scale. We hope that our final product will provide an authoritative summary of our current knowledge of the roentgen manifestations of tumors.

PHILIP J. HODES
Editor-in-Chief

Thomas Jefferson University Hospital

Editorial Advisory Committee

HARRY L. BERMAN   VINCENT P. COLLINS   E. RICHARD KING
LEO G. RIGLER   PHILIP RUBIN

Author's Preface

THOUGH one of the most prevalent sites of neoplasia and one of the more ideal regions for radiologic diagnosis, the female reproductive system has been sparingly examined by this method. This is in part due to over-reliance on physical diagnostic methods and laparotomy and is also due to widespread unfamiliarity with the contributions of radiology. The fact that precise histologic diagnosis by radiologic means is often thwarted by the extreme complexity of gynecologic pathology should not preclude our obtaining the useful information that is available. It is believed that whenever significant contributory knowledge about the presence, nature and extent of reproductive tract tumors can be gained by relatively riskless and inexpensive methods, we have the obligation to take advantage of them.

In this volume, honest effort has been made to emphasize the practical utility of certain means of radiologic diagnosis and to deemphasize the routine use of special studies. Radiologic study of the female reproductive tract has its limitations. These will be acknowledged and emphasized.

The reader will note that particular emphasis and space allocation have been given to some fairly commonplace entities and those conditions to which radiologic methods have a definite contribution to make. No effort has been made to illustrate countless "look-alikes" representing a great variety of tumors and tumorlike conditions for the sake of completeness. While much can and should be contributed to gynecologic tumor management by radiologic means, it is not, with a few rare exceptions, a substitute for skilled pathologic interpretation.

The most important contribution of radiology to the accurate diagnosis of tumors of the reproductive tract is to indicate or confirm the presence of any disease at all. Next most important is the designation of the site of involvement. In a few instances characteristic radiographic features will allow a precise diagnosis, but in most cases interpretation is based on gross pathologic outlines alone.

It has been my intention to extract from my personal experience, and that of others, the practical and promising radiologic approaches and the specific features which distinguish one entity from another. Winnowing the wheat from the chaff is a difficult and sometimes arbitrary task. As can be seen, I have drawn heavily on the work of others who have most generously shared their experience. Particularly important contributions to this volume have been made by Dr. Alfred Breit, Passau, West Germany; by Drs. Claes Rådberg and Ingmar Wickbom, Gothenberg, Sweden; Drs. R. A. L. Brewis and K. D. Bagshawe, London, England, and Dr. James J. McCort, San Jose, Calif. Without these contributions the volume would indeed have been incomplete. Additional case material has been provided by several others, to whom grateful acknowledgment is included with the illustrations they provided.

Without the skillful prodding and suggestions of our Editor-in-Chief, Philip Hodes, this volume would have been even further delayed in reaching print. If the volume fails to fulfill its intended purpose, it will not be the fault of Mr. William Cornwell and his staff at Eastman Kodak, who have provided superb photographic skills for the processing of these illustrations and who have permitted me to use several pelvic pneumograms from a previous publication in *Medical Radiography and Photography*.

G. MELVIN STEVENS

PART 1

Radiologic Techniques, 1

PART 2

The Uterus and Vagina, 21

PART 3

The Ovaries and Adnexa, 175

PART 4

Extrapelvic Tumor Extension and Recurrence, 311

Index, 337

Radiologic Techniques

Radiologic Techniques in Diagnosis

RADIOLOGIC INVESTIGATION of the female reproductive tract is accomplished primarily by (1) plain radiographic interpretation, (2) pelvic pneumography, (3) uterosalpingography, (4) pelvic arteriography, and (5) amniography (technique discussed on p. 118). Lymphangiography and pelvic venography are supplementary techniques utilized in the assessment of tumor extension or recurrence. The following techniques in conducting these investigations have been found practical and useful, though by no means the only way to "skin the cat."

PLAIN FILMS OF THE PELVIS

The suspicion of a reproductive tract tumor may originate with the patient's history or the physical findings, but not uncommonly the first evidence of a pelvic mass is observed on plain films of the pelvis. Of first importance is proper film exposure. To enhance the slight differences in radiodensity between water, fat and gas it is important that exposures be made in the low kilovolt range (65–75). The bladder must be completely emptied before radiography, and it is helpful if a cathartic or enema has caused the elimination of solid stool.

The outlines of the uterus and bladder are commonly, though not always, visible on plain roentgenograms (Fig. 1). One or both normal ovaries can occasionally be identified. When these organs enlarge, displacement of the normal ileal, cecal and rectosigmoid structures plus the primary density of the mass itself sometimes allow identification. Rarely the radiographic evidence of gas in a degenerating fibroid can be recognized, providing evidence of infection by a gas-forming organism.[1]

The presence of calcification, ossification, dental structure and fat within a mass has important diagnostic significance, generally indicating a benign dermoid cyst. On occasion a relative change in position of phleboliths in the pelvis will provide indirect evidence of an enlarging mass or infiltrative process, or the number and distribution of phleboliths may identify a pelvic hemangioma.[2] Oblique films may be important in recognizing radiographic

---

[1] Seaman, W. B., and Fleming, R. J.: Pneumatosis of pelvic viscera, Seminars Roentgenol. 4:202, 1969.

[2] Noonan, C. D.: Roentgen diagnosis of gynecologic disorders using conventional methods: Plain films, barium studies, pyelography, cystography, Seminars Roentgenol. 4:186, 1969; Primary and secondary malignancy of the female reproductive system, Radiol. Clin. North America 3:375, 1965.

signs of abnormality which are otherwise obscured by the sacrum and coccyx or gas and feces in the intestine. Proper interpretation of the evidence suggesting a mass is important both to avoid a false negative interpretation and to avoid false positive diagnoses which lead to expensive and anxiety-producing clarifying examinations.

The presence of intraperitoneal fluid in the pelvis and lower abdomen is recognized by ground-glass radiodensity in the areas where fluid has accumulated, effacement of the properitoneal fat lines and broadening of the flank stripe due to fluid interposed between the bowel and the abdominal wall. Depending on the position during filming, the flank stripe width will vary as more fluid shifts to the dependent side. In the upper abdomen, the hepatic angle and splenic angles are normally visible when the patient is supine. Ascitic fluid in this position compresses the relatively fluid extraperitoneal perivisceral fat pad and in addition anteriorly displaces the posterior aspect of the liver and spleen from the fat pad. The combination of these two occurrences causes the loss of these otherwise evident angles. Extraperitoneal fluid will also efface these angles, though the mechanism is different.[3] Numerous examples of the use of plain film diagnosis will be found in the following pages.

PELVIC PNEUMOGRAPHY

After a half-century of usage by physicians throughout the world pelvic pneumography has proved its practical usefulness and safety. It can be employed on an outpatient basis and involves only moderate costs and minimal risks for the patient. Wherever delineation of the gross outlines of the reproductive tract, the supporting ligaments and the peritoneal surfaces of the pelvis may be helpful in identifying the presence and the nature of a disease process, pelvic pneumography may be helpful. This is particularly true when bimanual pelvic examination is handicapped by various physical obstacles to satisfactory examination such as pelvic pain, virginal introitus, thick abdominal musculature, obesity or confusion due to adjacent urinary or alimentary tract structures or disease. Of the special radiographic procedures available in gynecologic diagnosis, pelvic pneumography has the broadest applicability and requires the most common use.

PNEUMOPERITONEUM TECHNIQUE.—Greater detail than seems appropriate here, regarding the technique of inducing pneumoperitoneum, may be found in an earlier publication.[4]

---

[3] Whalen, J. P.; Berne, A. S., and Riemenschneider, P. A.: The extraperitoneal perivascular fat pad: Its role in the roentgenologic visualization of abdominal organs, Radiology 92:466, 1969; The extraperitoneal fat pad: II. Roentgen interpretation of pathological alterations, *Ibid.*, p. 473.

[4] Stevens, G. M.; Weigen, J. F., and Lee, R. S.: Pelvic pneumography, M. Radiog. & Photog. 42:82, 1966.

Choice of gas.—Both carbon dioxide and nitrous oxide have been used as gaseous contrast agents, though the latter is preferred for two reasons. (1) Its solubility in blood and water is somewhat less than that of carbon dioxide, thus providing adequate time for standard radiography, supplementary views and repeat films if necessary while retaining the advantage of a high solubility which limits the possibility of gas embolism and allows rapid resorption after the procedure. (2) Nitrous oxide, in our experience, has caused significantly less peritoneal pain than carbon dioxide.

Patient preparation.—Omission of the meal prior to pelvic pneumography, a thorough cleansing enema of the rectum and sigmoid and complete bladder emptying immediately prior to the procedure constitute the necessary preparation. The preliminary film is taken to assure the thoroughness of the preparation and adequate exposure. Allowance must be made for the marked increase in pelvic radiolucency following pneumatization. The bladder should be emptied after the preliminary film and immediately before gas is introduced in order to avoid superimposition of the pelvic organs by the urine-filled bladder.

Gas instillation.—Gas can be introduced by transtubal insufflation if the tubes are known to be patent, but in general if pelvic examination has previously been conducted by the referring physician it is easier for the patient and radiologist alike to instill gas by way of transabdominal needle puncture. For this purpose, a site is selected in the left upper quadrant lateral to the rectus abdominus muscle and slightly below the costal margin. The skin is cleansed with an antiseptic solution and skin anesthesia is induced by use of a dermal needle. A no. 20, 1½–3 in. needle (depending on the abdominal wall thickness) is attached to the local anesthesia syringe and the anesthetic agent is administered to the level of the peritoneum. The peritoneum is then penetrated, generally announced by a slight "pop through" sensation and slight pain. After aspiration to avoid intravascular injection, a small amount of residual anesthetic is then injected; the diminished resistance to injection can be recognized when the needle tip is in the peritoneal space. This fact is confirmed when a small amount of air is then injected with hardly any resistance and cannot be retrieved in the syringe on aspiration. The pneumoperitoneum apparatus is then connected and approximately 1200 cc of nitrous oxide is introduced. This procedure is essentially painless. If pain develops, particularly at the site of injection or in the flank or inguinal region, this may be taken as nearly certain evidence of extraperitoneal inflation and the position of the needle tip must be adjusted. Any pneumoperitoneum apparatus which allows a controlled flow and measured volume of gas without contamination from atmospheric air is satisfactory.

After removal of the needle the patient is turned to a prone position and the head of the tilt table is inverted 45°. By placing the hands beneath the abdomen, the radiologist can "jiggle" the abdominal viscera cephalad, allowing the volume of nitrous oxide to rise to fill the pelvis.

Radiographic procedure.—All films are taken in the inverted position, as shown in Figure 2. The exposure is centered over the coccyx and the first film is made with the central ray perpendicular to the floor (cephalad at an angle of 45°). Subsequent films are taken with the tube angled 10° and 20° caudad (in effect, 55° and 65° angles between patient and central ray). By shifting and angling the tube and by leaving the film tray in position, the latter two exposures constitute a stereoscopic pair. Additional 30° right and left anterior oblique films with the tube angled 10° caudad complete the routine. On occasion, cross-table horizontal beam films are made with the patient lying prone. The normal anatomy demonstrated by this procedure is seen in Figure 3. It should be noted that *all of the pelvic pneumograms are presented in reverse; in other words, the reader looks at the films as though the patient were lying supine, although they were taken in postero-anterior position.*

After-care.—Because of some residual discomfort from the referred pain of subdiaphragmatic gas, the patient ordinarily prefers to recline for 30–45 minutes before going home or returning to her hospital room. Approximately 75% of the gas is absorbed within 2 hours, and if the study is performed in the afternoon there is generally insignificant or no residual discomfort the following morning.

UTEROSALPINGOGRAPHY

The procedure for uterosalpingography has been fairly well standardized.[5] The cervix is inspected by means of a bivalve side-opening speculum, after which the upper vagina and cervix are cleansed with germicidal detergent and antiseptic solution. Although we have employed a tenaculum to secure the cervix and a cannula to introduce the contrast medium, there is a good case for the use of a vacuum cannula, unless the cervix is badly deformed or lacerated. Standard and large-size rubber acorn tips for the cannula tip should be available for proper occlusion of the external os during retrograde filling. Only a short length of cannula tip should extend beyond the rubber acorn so that the cervical canal and the endometrial detail are not obscured; there is less chance of perforation as well.

---

[5] Dalsace, J., and Garcia-Calderon, J.: *Gynecologic Radiography* (New York: Paul B. Hoeber, Inc., 1959). Rozin, S.: *Uterosalpingography in Gynecology* (Springfield, Ill.: Charles C Thomas, Publisher, 1965).

A syringe containing the contrast medium is attached to the cannula and all air bubbles are evacuated. The system should then be closed by a stopcock. After the cannula is securely seated in the cervix, the speculum is removed to minimize discomfort and eliminate obscuration. By means of a fractional filling technique with interval films made under image amplifier guidance, the contrast injection is completed. Spot films are taken in the supine and oblique positions, and at times in the prone position as well. Film detail is improved by bringing the spot film device into contact with the patient. Effort should be made to straighten an acutely flexed uterus by gentle traction on the tenaculum while cannula occlusion is maintained by gentle pressure in the opposite direction. From 4–10 cc of contrast medium is usually required for adequate filling of the uterus and tubes. The contrast medium generally flows readily from the fimbriated end of the tube into the peritoneal cavity. Occasionally delay of retrograde flow at the cornu is due to tubal spasm. This can be overcome by persistent gentle pressure in some, and in others by premedication with a smooth muscle relaxant such as Vasodilin.

Most radiologists strongly prefer to use a water-soluble contrast medium in order to (1) avoid oil embolization, (2) diminish the likelihood of granuloma formation, (3) improve the miscibility of contrast and uterine secretions, and (4) diminish radiation exposure by more rapid filling with less viscous contrast. When a premenopausal patient is to be examined it is prudent to conduct the investigation in the preovulatory phase to avoid irradiation of an unsuspected early pregnancy. Acute pelvic infections and active bleeding constitute contraindications to uterosalpingography.

Normal anatomy as demonstrated by uterosalpingography is illustrated in Figure 4.

PELVIC ANGIOGRAPHY

High hopes for the diagnostic contribution of this procedure have been held for many years and enthusiastic reports have been made by numerous authors. The cumulative experience in pelvic angiography since Borell et al.[6] initiated the use of catheter arteriography in 1952, however, illuminates one reality which has not been sufficiently stressed. While abnormal vascular patterns can be recognized in a very high portion of reproductive tract tumors, particularly with selective hypogastric arteriography, the features are generally neither distinctive nor constant enough to identify most types of

[6] Borell, U.; Fernström, I.; Lindblom, K., and Westman, A.: The diagnostic value of arteriography of the iliac artery in gynecology and obstetrics, Acta Radiol. (diag.) 38:247, 1952.

tumor. One must contend with the extreme complexity and subtlety of many reproductive tract tumors, particularly those of the ovary.

Since reliable distinction between most benign and malignant tumors cannot be made, the practical usefulness of arteriography is limited to a few special categories: (1) Patients in whom distinction between uterine and adnexal disease is important, particularly when the size of the mass or adhesions prevents satisfactory pneumatization of the pelvis for pelvic pneumography or culdoscopy. (2) Staging and assessment of tumor recurrence in carcinoma of the cervix. (3) Selected problem cases of trophoblastic tumors.

Certain arteriographic signs of abnormality have, however, been recognized as highly reliable. Among these is separation of the junctions of the parametrial and marginal segments of the uterine artery, which gives reliable evidence of uterine enlargement. Likewise, lateral displacement of the marginal arteries indicates enlargement of the uterus. Intramural tumors are indicated by obstruction, deflection and distortion of the intramural arcades as well as by the presence of tumor vessels. Tumor vessels in the parametrium are less easily recognized because of their usual diminutive size, but enlargement of the ovarian or uterine adnexal arteries, the presence of tumor vessels and the deflection of normal vasculature all provide reliable signs of abnormality. Examples of the application of arteriography and tumor diagnosis emphasizing the above three categories will be found throughout this volume.

TECHNIQUE.—Pelvic angiography by catheterization technique was described most completely in the monograph by Fernström,[7] and since that time little has been added except for the employment of selective hypogastric artery injections in appropriate situations.[8] Preparation includes catharsis and introduction of an indwelling catheter, the latter to avoid accumulation of contrast medium in the bladder during arteriography.

Catheters are introduced by the Seldinger technique from a retrograde approach in the femoral artery. For intra-aortic injection a Teflon or polyethylene catheter of approximately 0.062 in. internal diameter and 60 cm length is used. Most radiologists prefer several side holes near the catheter tip and the use of a tip occluder to prevent retrograde filling of abdominal visceral tributaries, particularly the inferior mesenteric artery. The catheter tip is placed just above the aortic bifurcation for bilateral uterine artery

---

[7] Fernström, I.: Arteriography of the uterine artery: Its value in the diagnosis of uterine fibroma, tubal pregnancy, adnexal tumor, and placental site localization in cases of intrauterine pregnancy, Acta Radiol. (diag.), supp. 122, p. 128, 1955.
[8] Altemus, R.: Differentiating uterine and extrauterine masses by bilateral selective hypogastric arteriography, Radiology 92:1020, 1969. For a review of pelvic angiography see Rådberg, C., and Wickbom, I.: Pelvic angiography and pneumoperitoneum in the diagnosis of gynecologic lesions, Acta Radiol. (diag.) 6:133, 1967.

filling and at the level of the third lumbar segment for inclusion of the ovarian arteries. Sixty cubic centimeters of 75% sodium or meglumine diatrizoate solution is used when injected in the aorta and 12–20 cc of 50–60% contrast in each hypogastric artery when injected selectively. In the latter case a sharply flexed Teflon or polyethylene catheter must be engaged in each hypogastric artery, generally by bilateral retrograde femoral approach. Contrast should be injected at a rate of 15 cc per second for intra-aortic injection and at the rate of 12–15 cc per second when injected selectively using a Y connector. Films are exposed starting near the end of injection at the rate of two per second for 4 seconds, then one per second for the remainder to cover a total period of 12–15 seconds. Generally only posteroanterior films are necessary, but occasionally oblique films may be helpful. Most experienced angiographers advocate the use of bilateral femoral artery compression during injection and filming in order to maximize concentration in the pelvic vessels. Meticulous technique during the procedure and in postarteriography care will prevent all but rare complications, which largely consist of thrombosis, bleeding and embolization.

PELVIC ARTERIAL ANATOMY.—The origin of the uterine artery is generally obscured by the other pelvic vessels, but it most often arises from the internal iliac artery and occasionally by a common trunk with the internal pudendal or vaginal arteries (Fig. 5). It passes caudad along the pelvic wall to its transverse course in the parametrium, then divides into the larger cephalad-coursing uterine marginal branch and the smaller caudad-directed cervical vaginal branch. The marginal portion in turn gives off spiral intramural tributaries which produce arcades anastomosing with their counterparts on the opposite side. Near the fundus a branch courses medially to the fundus, and a larger tributary constituting the adnexal branch passes laterally to the ovary, fallopian tube and broad ligament.

The ovarian arteries originate from the anterior aspect of the abdominal aorta below the renal arteries and pass down in a tortuous course through the infundibulopelvic ligaments to the ovary. They contribute in varying degrees to the blood supply of the ovary and adnexal structures. The caliber of uterine and ovarian arteries will depend on the patient's age, being most prominent in the active reproductive period and atrophying after menopause. Uterine and ovarian vein tributaries are seldom seen with the flush type arterial injection and are rarely of diagnostic value in selective examinations in gynecologic problems unless there is arterial-venous shunting.

Figure 1.—Plain film of a normal pelvis.

A, anteroposterior plain film of pelvic soft tissues.

B, drawing of **A,** delineating uterus (**a**), ovaries (**b**), urinary bladder (**c**), iliopsoas muscle (**d**).

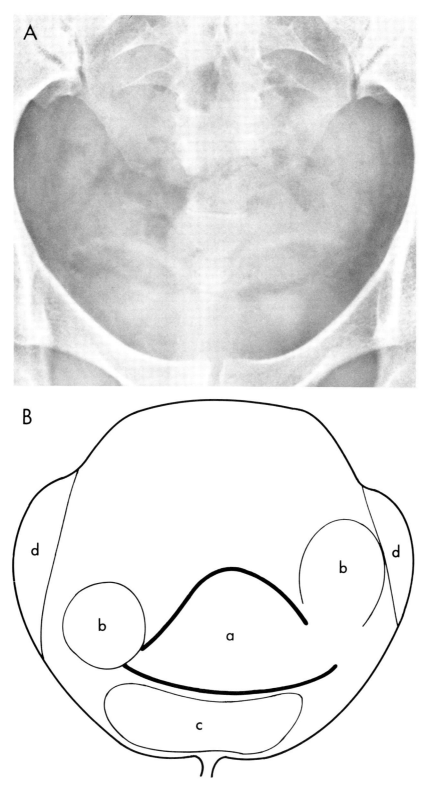

Figure 1 · Plain Film of Pelvis: Normal Anatomy / 11

Figure 2.—Pelvic pneumography: technique.

Positioning of the patient and angulation of the x-ray beam for making (**A**) posteroanterior, and (**B**) prone oblique pelvic pneumograms.

Figures 2 and 3 from Stevens, G. M.; Weigen, J. F., and Lee, R. S.: M. Radiog. & Photog. 42:82, 1966.

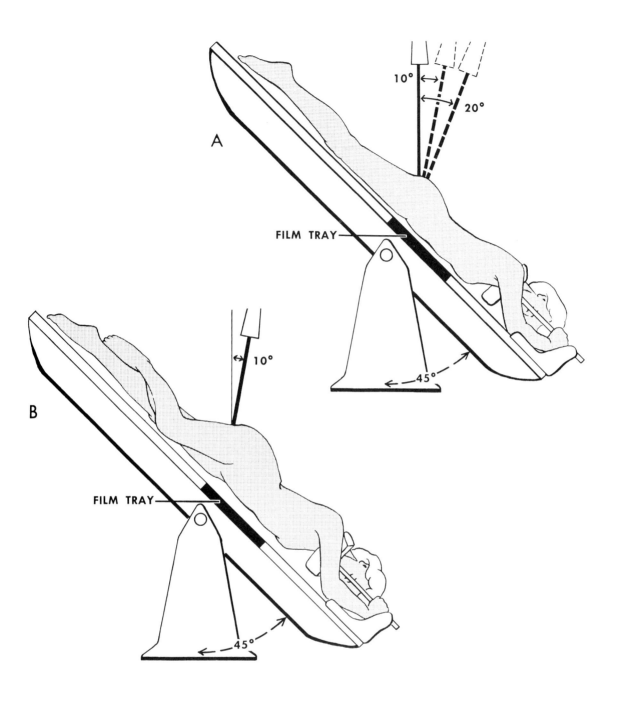

Figure 2 · Pelvic Pneumography: Technique / 13

Figure 3.—Pelvic pneumography; normal anatomy.

A, posteroanterior exposure; position as in Figure 2, *A*.

B, right prone oblique position; orientation as in Figure 2, *B*.

C, lateral exposure; position as in Figure 2, *A*.

1, rectum
2, sigmoid colon
3, cul-de-sac of Douglas (rectouterine pouch)
4, uterosacral ligament
5, ureter
6, infundibulopelvic ligament
7, fallopian tube
8, ovary
9, broad ligament
10, ovarian ligament
11, round ligament
12, uterine fundus
13, uterine isthmus
14, intergluteal crease
15, urinary bladder
16, transverse vesical fold
17, uterovesical pouch

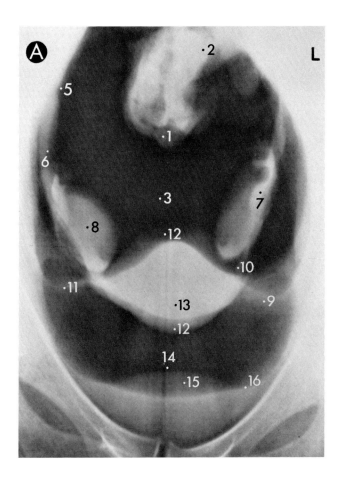

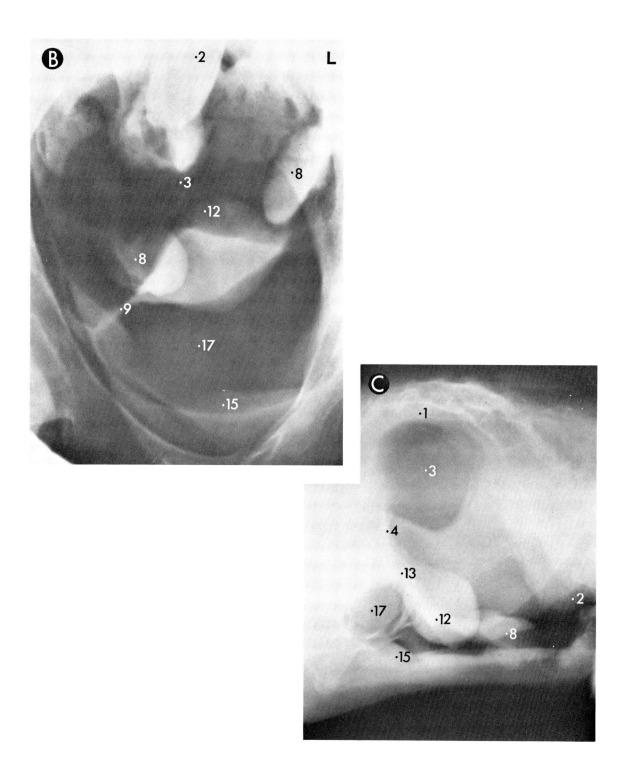

Figure 3 · Pelvic Pneumography: Normal Anatomy / 15

Figure 4.—Hysterosalpingography; normal anatomy.

A, left posterior oblique exposure; normal anteflexed uterus. Uterine fundus (**a**), cervical canal (**b**), isthmus of fallopian tube (**c**), ampulla (**d**), fimbriated end of tube (**e**).

B, right posterior oblique position.

C, anteroposterior postevacuation film. Residual contrast delineates uterus (**a**) and ovaries (**arrows**).

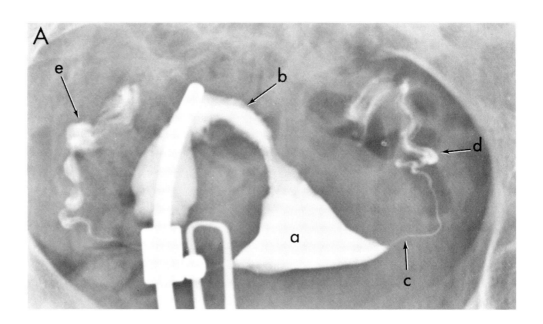

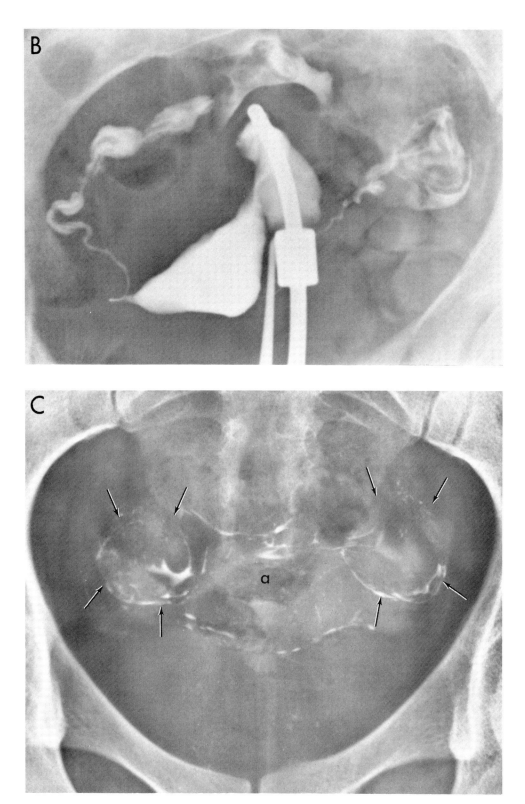

Figure 4 · Hysterosalpingography: Normal Anatomy / 17

Figure 5.—Pelvic arteriography; normal anatomy.

A, normal pelvic arteriogram, arterial phase, 1½ seconds after completion of the injection.

B, drawing of **A,** delineating external iliac artery (**1**); internal (hypogastric) iliac artery (**2**); inferior gluteal artery (**3**); uterine artery (**4**); cervical vaginal branch of uterine artery (**5**); vaginal branch of internal pudendal artery (**6**); internal pudendal artery (**7**); obturator artery (**8**).

C, 3 seconds after completion of injection (late arterial and precapillary phase): right uterine artery still filled; beginning visualization of intramural tributaries. The uterus is somewhat enlarged.

D, 4 seconds after completion of injection (uterine intramural phase): beginning visualization of bladder. The right ovarian artery is filled (**arrow**).

Figure 5, courtesy of Dr. A. Breit, Passau, W. Germany.

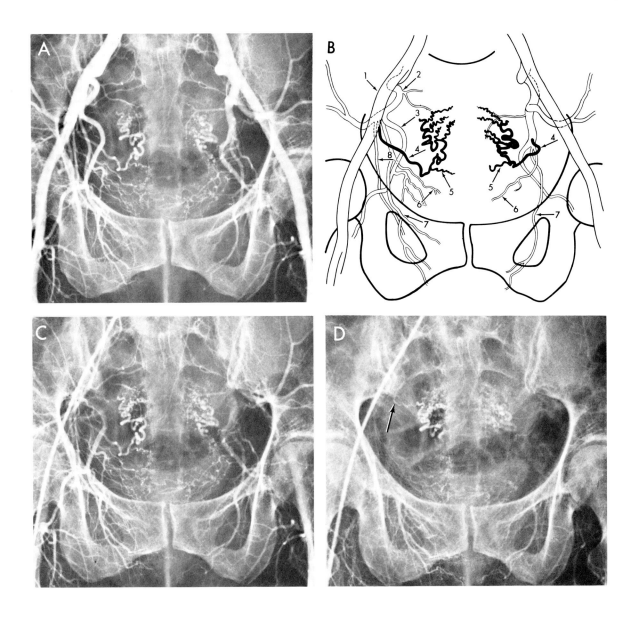

Figure 5 · Pelvic Arteriography: Normal Anatomy / 19

PART 2

The Uterus and Vagina

Uterine Tumors and Tumorlike Conditions

MENTION SHOULD BE MADE of the more common entities which one might encounter in radiologic investigation of the uterus. No attempt is made to provide a detailed discussion nor even a comprehensive list of the varied tumors or tumorlike conditions which involve the uterus. Detailed descriptions are available in standard texts.[1–4]

ENDOMETRIAL HYPERPLASIA.—Endometrial hyperplasia is characterized by voluminous redundant polypoid folds which may be localized but is most often diffuse. This process appears to be stimulated by prolonged or unopposed estrogen stimulation and is therefore found in patients who are receiving therapeutic estrogen or those with Stein-Levinthal syndrome, for example. Hyperplasia generally stops abruptly at the internal os since the endocervical mucosa is less responsive to hormone influence (Fig. 14, *B*). This feature might be of some assistance in distinguishing hyperplasia from carcinoma, where the tumor recognizes no such demarcation. At times the histologic differentiation of endometrial hyperplasia from well-differentiated endometrial carcinoma is very difficult.

ENDOMETRIAL POLYPS.—Sessile or pedunculated mucosal projections composed of hyperplastic, hypertrophied or neoplastic glands and stroma of the endometrium are recognized as polyps (Fig. 28). They may be single or multiple and vary from a tiny size to 10 or 12 cm in diameter. Most are found at or near the time of menopause and they come to the patient's attention by ulcerating or becoming irritated and bleeding. Approximately 10% of patients who have endometrial polyps in the postmenopausal period also have endometrial carcinoma and 30% of patients with endometrial carcinoma have had polyps removed previously,[1] thus showing a strong relationship between these two entities. It is not uncommon that polyps will escape detection during curettage.

ENDOMETRIAL CARCINOMA.—Occurring most commonly in postmenopausal women (average age 57), these tumors, which are generally friable

---

[1] Kraus, F. T.: *Gynecologic Pathology* (St. Louis: C. V. Mosby Company, 1967).

[2] Anderson, W. A. D. (ed.): *Pathology* (5th ed.; St. Louis: C. V. Mosby Company, 1966), Vol. 2.

[3] Novak, E. R., and Woodruff, J. D.: *Novak's Gynecologic and Obstetric Pathology: With Clinical and Endocrine Relations* (6th ed.; Philadelphia: W. B. Saunders Company, 1967).

[4] Hertig, A. T., and Gore, H.: "Tumors of the Female Sex Organs: Part 2. Tumors of the Vulva, Vagina and Uterus," in Armed Forces Institute of Pathology *Atlas of Tumor Pathology*, Sec. IX, Fasc. 33, Pt. 2 (1960) and Supplement (1968).

and often ulcerated and necrotic, make their presence known by vaginal bleeding. They may be focal or diffuse but are generally localized. In the former type the entire interior of the uterus is sometimes involved, and the tumor may extend into the cervical canal (Fig. 32, *A*). In advanced cases the disease may extend to the peritoneum and in so doing produce a gross uterine enlargement and occasionally small tumor nodules on the uterine surface. More often, however, the uterus is not grossly enlarged. The relatively favorable survival with proper management requires that this tumor be accurately recognized and promptly treated.

Because of the accessibility of endometrial carcinoma for diagnosis by curettage and biopsy, the role of radiology in tumor diagnosis has been limited. The practical role of hysterography as described by Norman is found on pages 74 ff.

Mixed Mesodermal Tumors; Sarcoma of the Endometrium.—The average age of patients with this uncommon tumor is the mid-sixties (see Fig. 39). Grossly it consists of pink polypoid excrescences often protruding into the cervical os or vagina. Mixed mesodermal tumors are generally highly malignant. Pure sarcomas of the endometrium are commonly of low grade and afflict younger women. Pathologists not infrequently have considerable difficulty in distinguishing between benign and malignant varieties of these tumors.

Myometrial Tumors.—*Adenomyosis.*—The presence of endometrial glands and stroma within the myometrium characterizes adenomyosis. Uterine muscular hypertrophy is an associated feature in most cases. This process is particularly inclined to involve the posterior uterine wall producing moderate globe-shaped uterine enlargement. Asymmetrical involvement of the uterine wall by adenomyosis is uncommon. On occasion, lateral humps near the cornua are seen.

Colicky dysmenorrhea and abnormal uterine bleeding are typical symptoms. The pelvic pain may be referred to the lower rectum and sacrococcygeal area. Adenomyosis and endometriosis have been found to coexist (Fig. 70) in 15-40% of patients, depending on the author reporting. Likewise, adenomyosis and myomas often coexist.

Myomas (Fibroids).—See pages 25 ff.

Hemangiopericytoma.—This tumor is rare in the myometrium and is generally found by serendipity on removal of the uterus for fibroids. Although generally benign, it is malignant on occasion. It is generally discrete and is comprised of moderately soft yellow or gray nodules.

Other rare tumors include lipomas of the myometrium, which would theoretically be recognizable by their radiolucency, and cysts of the myometrium, which are generally of müllerian duct origin.

TROPHOBLASTIC TUMORS.—See pages 118 ff.

VAGINAL TUMORS.—Since these tumors are readily accessible for biopsy, radiologic diagnosis has played only a very small role in their management. Sarcoma botryoides (Figs. 66–68) is one exception since it is seen most commonly in infants and arises from the upper vagina or cervix and produces grayish red polypoid masses which may fill the vagina. Because of the difficulties of examining so small a child and ascertaining the extent of involvement, vaginography and opacification of the adjacent bladder and colon may be helpful. Bleeding generally signals the presence of such a tumor. Because of its benign histologic appearance it is often underdiagnosed, but the patient's age, gross appearance of the tumor and history of vaginal bleeding are nearly diagnostic in themselves.

Other tumors of epithelial or mesodermal origin arising in the vagina in adults are managed without the assistance of diagnostic radiology.

Uterine Leiomyoma (Fibroid)

Uterine leiomyomas (fibroids) are the commonest tumors of the female reproductive tract, and are particularly common among Negroes. About 20% of women over 30 have one or more fibroids; thus they may be encountered at almost any age after puberty. Because of diminished estrogen effect they involute following the menopause. Most fibroids are subserous or intramural; about 5% are submucosal. The submucosal variety rarely calcify; the others frequently do. Both subserous and submucous fibroids may become pedunculated and create confusing clinical findings and curettement problems requiring radiologic diagnostic assistance. Since fibroids vary from a few millimeters to over 100 lb., size has no practical diagnostic significance. On occasion a fibroid occurs in the broad ligament (Figs. 10, 18 and 22) or on the cervix.

Fibroid calcification results from necrosis or degeneration of the myomatous and fibrous elements and may assume a great variety of patterns. Some of the patterns are characteristic and virtually pathognomonic; others are very difficult to recognize (Figs. 12, 8, *B* and 24, *B*). Initial punctate or irregular scattered calcifications may multiply, enlarge and coalesce to produce flakes and aggregates of calcification; less commonly, a peripheral rim of calcification is observed (Figs. 9, *A*, 19 and 24, *B*). Calcific deposition is a slow process requiring many years in most instances. Rarely, metaplasia is responsible for the deposition of osseous material. Rather sparse vascularity characterizes most fibroid tumors (Figs. 25, 27).

The type and variety of radiographic features are generously illustrated here due to the frequency of fibroids and the practical importance of their accurate recognition.

Fortunately sarcomatous degeneration of uterine fibroid is rare since this entity is generally only recognized by microscopic examination. There is no practical way, with present techniques, to diagnose malignant transformation by radiologic methods.

Figure 6.—Varied calcific patterns in uterine fibroids.

A, anteroposterior projection: Very large, heavily calcified fibroid filling the pelvis of a patient, 56; known to be present and calcified for 15 years.

B, anteroposterior projection: Multiple heavily calcified fibroids in a woman of 77.

C, anteroposterior view: A small round calcific aggregate present in a right pelvic fibroid in a woman age 57.

D (same patient as in **C,** 12 years later), anteroposterior view: More densely calcific fibroid but no growth in size in this postmenopausal period.

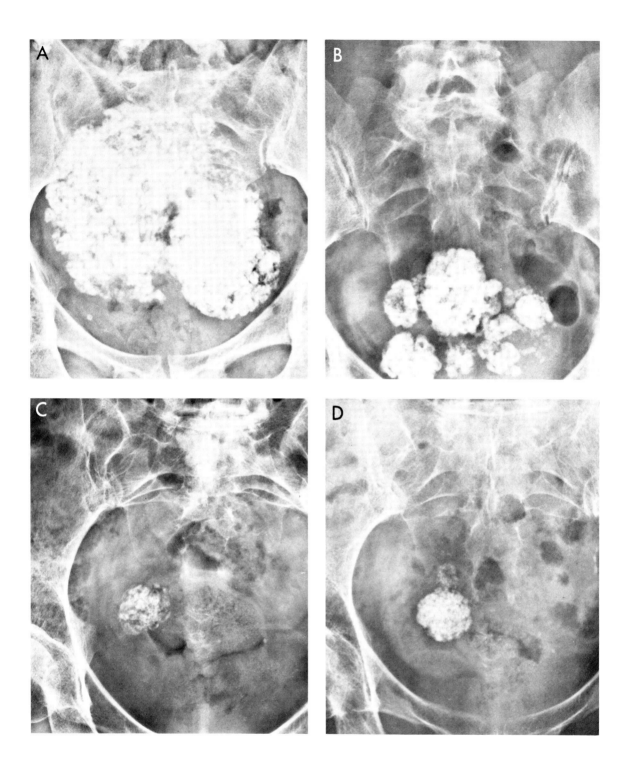

Figure 6 · Fibroids: Calcific Patterns / 27

Figure 7.—Massive uterine fibroids.

A, anteroposterior exposure: Enormous central abdominal mass containing small area of calcification in left upper quadrant. The colon is extrinsically displaced.

B, anteroposterior view: Demonstrating that the abdominal mass is extrinsic to urinary tract. Note delineation between mass and bladder (**arrows**).

C, lateral view of abdomen: Demonstrating the anterior location of mass.

D, oblique view: Delineating massive uterine fibroids. Note small calcification in the superior pole of the mass.

A 44-year-old woman entered the hospital with a history of recent menorrhagia and slowly progressive abdominal swelling for four years. Her general health had been excellent. A huge abdominal mass was palpable. Radiographic examination suggested reproductive tract origin. At surgery the uterus was enlarged to 30 × 20 cm by innumerable fibroids, the largest of which was 11 cm in diameter.

Comment: The supravesical, anterior central abdominal location of the mass strongly suggests its origin in the reproductive tract, but the size of the mass is more consistent with ovarian cyst or tumor. The uterine fibroids are exceptionally large in this case.

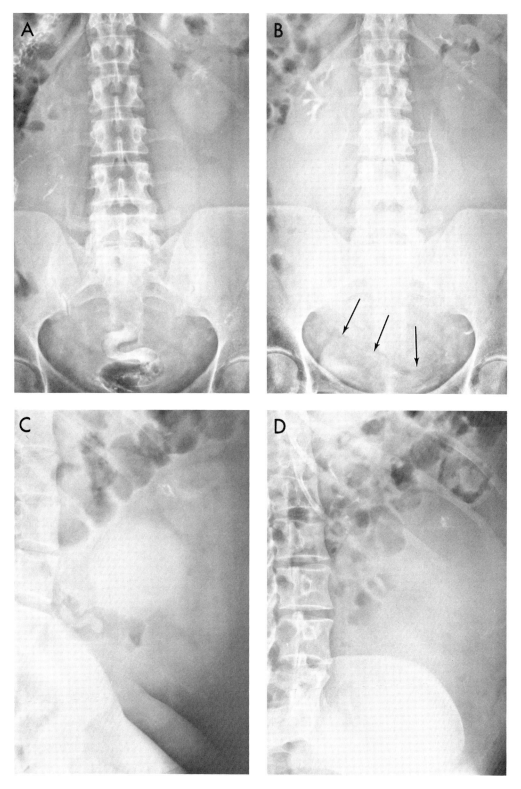

Figure 7 · Massive Uterine Fibroids / 29

Figure 8.—Varied calcific patterns in uterine fibroids.

A, anteroposterior projection: Mottled eggshell calcification in periphery of a fibroid. The patient, age 59, had metastatic carcinoma of the breast and a pelvic mass.

B, anteroposterior view: Small plaques and aggregates of faint calcification in a fibroid in the right pelvis (**arrows**) in a woman of 60.

C, anteroposterior view: Scattered and coalesced aggregations of dense calcification in a large fibroid in a patient age 57.

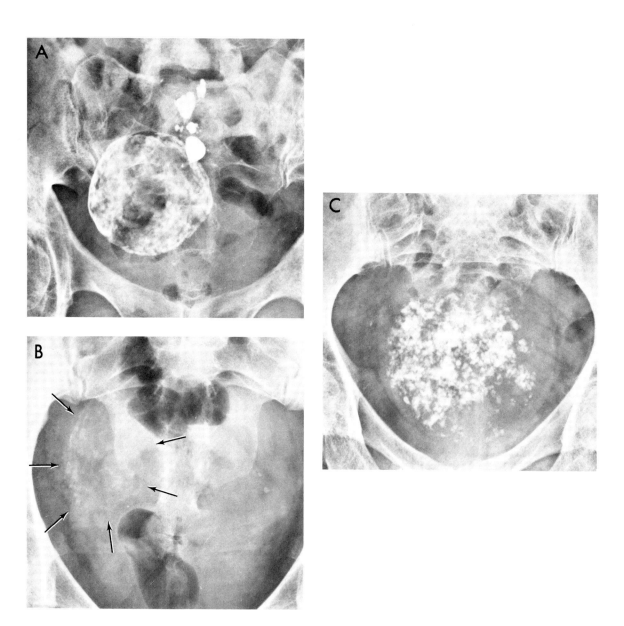

Figure 8 · Fibroids: Calcific Patterns / 31

Figure 9.—Uterine fibroids: pelvic pneumography (posteroanterior projections).

A, Small, oval subserous fibroid with eggshell calcification (**a**). An uncalcified small fibroid of the isthmus is partially obscured by the fundus (**b**). The slightly enlarged left ovary (**c**) is cystic.

The patient, 35, had recent onset of posterior pelvic pain. The two small posterior fibroids seen here were resected by posterior colpotomy, with relief of symptoms. The calcified fibroid was infarcted.

B, Uterus (**b**) showing diffuse moderate enlargement with lobular contour due to multiple small intramural fibroids; normal ovaries (**c**).

This 32-year-old, gravida II patient had lower abdominal tenderness and an occasional sensation of a pelvic mass. Pelvic examination was inconclusive.

C, Enlarged posterior uterine fundus due to fibroid (**b**); normal right ovary (**c**); slightly cystic left ovary (**d**); sigmoid colon (**e**).

This unmarried, virginal woman, 36, had had midcycle (ovulatory) pain for three years, with accompanying extremely painful bowel movements. Enovid gave relief but had unacceptable side effects. Pelvic examination was believed normal but was technically difficult. At surgery the fibroid measured 6 × 4.5 cm; the ovaries were normal and no endometriosis was found.

D, Oval, pedunculated subserous fibroid attached to the right anterior uterine surface (**b**).

Lower abdominal intermittent pain and dysmenorrhea were the principal complaints of this 40-year-old woman. Moderate obesity and a virginal introitus handicapped pelvic examination. The uterus was believed to be normal. The fibroid identified on the pneumogram was surgically removed.

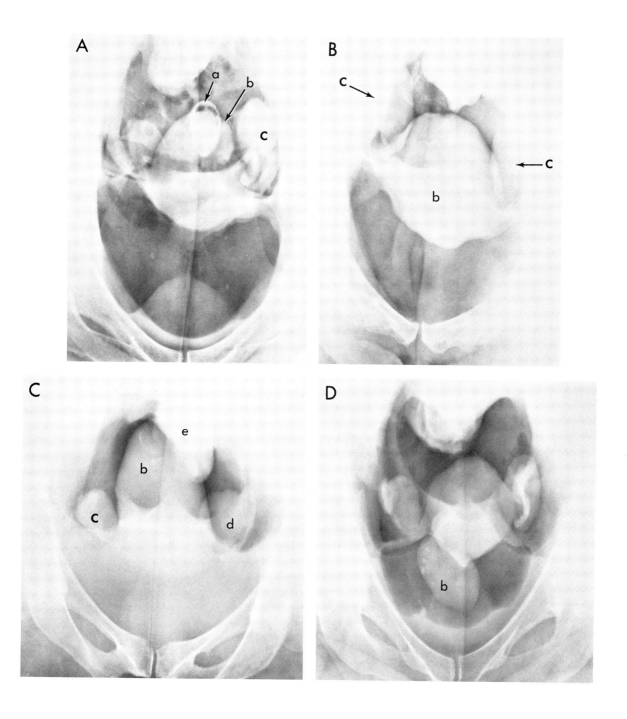

Figure 9 · Fibroids: Pelvic Pneumography / 33

Figure 10.—Uncalcified intraligamentous uterine fibroid.

A, anteroposterior projection: A large uncalcified intraligamentous fibroid tumor produces homogeneous density (**arrows**) arising above the bladder. Note perivesical fat demarcation (**a**).

B, excretory urogram: Establishing the extravesical origin of the mass. Both kidneys functioned adequately, though there was bilateral lower ureteral extrinsic pressure.

The patient, age 47, had a history of recent irregular menses, slight menorrhagia, intermenstrual spotting, urinary frequency and urgency. A large central pelvic mass was palpable. At surgery a 12 × 16 cm intraligamentous fibroid, moderately cystic ovaries and paraovarian cysts were removed.

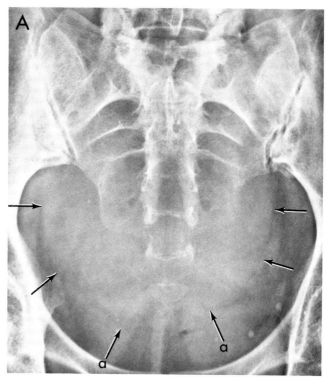

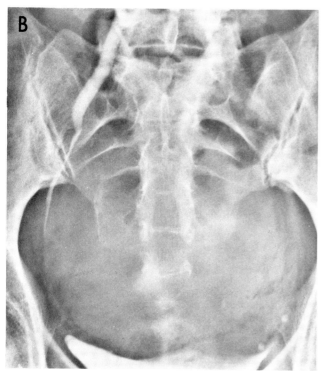

Figure 10 · Uncalcified Intraligamentous Fibroid / 35

Figure 11.—Calcified posterior uterine fibroids.

A, anteroposterior projection: Showing mottled, dense calcific clumps characterizing fibroids.

B, lateral projection: Demonstrating the posterior location of the calcified fibroids, which explains the difficulty experienced in performing sigmoidoscopy.

The patient, 76 years old, had a routine pelvic examination as part of a preoperative examination prior to a radical mastectomy. Firm, mobile uterine fibroids were palpable. She had been told 20 years previously that uterine fibroids were present.

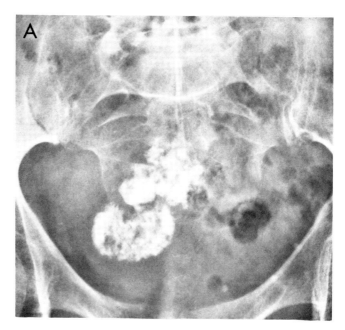

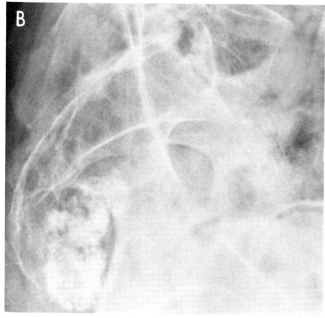

Figure 11 · Calcified Posterior Fibroids / 37

Figure 12.—Punctate fibroid calcifications.

A, anteroposterior excretory urogram: Showing uterine fibroids with punctate (**a**) and small aggregated (**b**) calcifications simulating ovarian psammomatous calcifications in the pelvis.

B, radiograph of sliced uterine surgical specimen: Showing calcific pattern in fibroids.

This 63-year-old virginal patient had a pelvic mass discovered incidental to investigation of *Escherichia coli* cystitis which had produced gross hematuria. Results of the initial pelvic examination were negative, but pelvic masses were detected after the urogram showed pelvic tumor and punctate calcifications suggesting psammoma bodies. A 5 cm cyst of the right ovary, a 7 cm solid thecoma of the left ovary and multiple uterine fibroids were discovered at surgery.

Comment: In reality these calcifications are more coarse and more widely separated than in psammoma bodies.

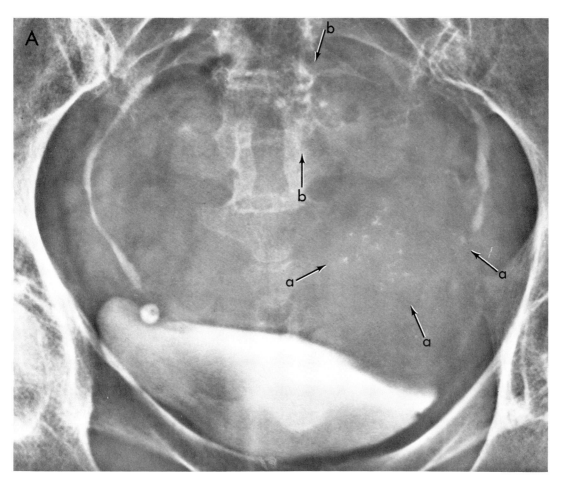

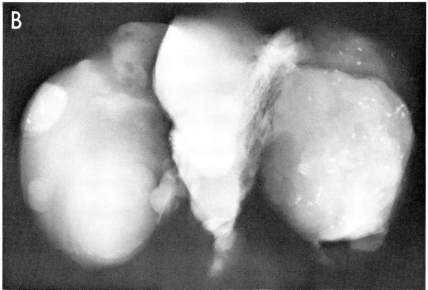

Figure 12 · Punctate Fibroid Calcifications / 39

Figure 13.—Fibroids: pelvic pneumography.

A, posteroanterior projection: Showing globular uterine enlargement due to intramural fibroids (**a**), normal ovaries (**b**) and bladder (**c**).

B, left anterior oblique projection: Showing calcified fibroids in the fundus (**a**). Ovaries (**b**); bladder (**c**).

A 64-year-old nulliparous widow had a history of recurrent right lower quadrant pain. Three physicians, including a gynecology consultant, believed a mass was present in the right pelvis. The gynecologist could palpate fibroid enlargement of the uterus as well. Cervical cytology was normal. Pelvic pneumography revealed no mass other than fibroid enlargement of the uterus. Surgery verified the radiologic interpretation and, when the uterus was opened, revealed an unsuspected small, well-differentiated endometrial carcinoma.

C, posteroanterior projection, with tube perpendicular to the floor: Demonstrating a bilobular mass comprised of enlargement of the uterine fundus containing mutiple small uncalcified fibroids (**a**) and large subserosal pedunculated fibroid (**d**). Left ovary (**b**).

D, posteroanterior projection, with 20° caudad angle of tube: Showing fibroid enlargement of the uterus (**a**), large pedunculated fibroid attached to the left anterior aspect of the uterus (**d**). Right round ligament (**e**); broad ligaments (**f**).

A gravida VI woman, age 52, was told she had uterine fibroids four years earlier, when menses were normal. Recent development of heavy menstruation with considerable clot formation led her to seek medical advice. The gynecologist suspected uterine fibroids, but adnexal examination was not conclusive. Surgery revealed multiple fibroids, including a large subserosal, partially pedunculated one arising from the left anterior aspect of the uterus; hysterectomy was performed.

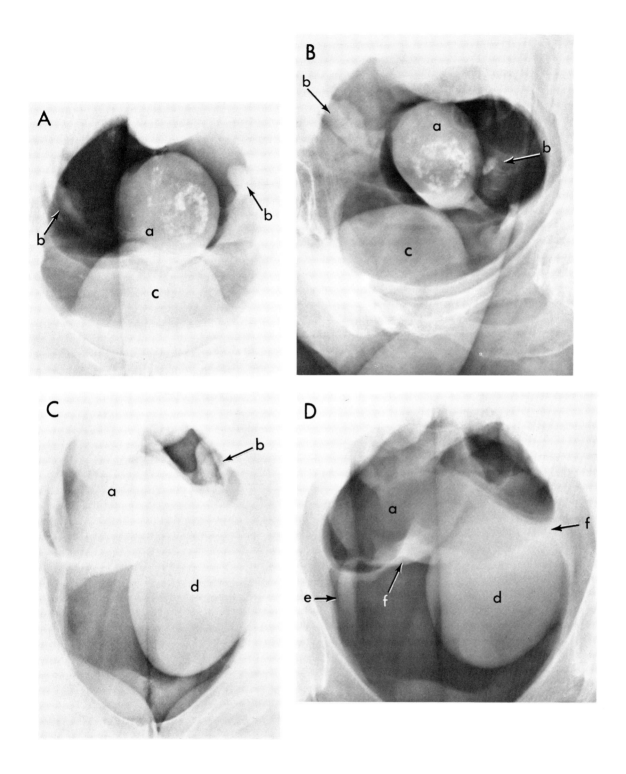

Figure 13 · Fibroids: Pelvic Pneumography / 41

Figure 14.—Large uterine fibroid in a young woman.

A, pelvic pneumogram, posteroanterior projection: Illustrating marked enlargement of the uterus (**a**), moderately enlarged right ovary (**b**) and normal left ovary (**c**).

B, uterosalpingogram, anteroposterior view: Outlining gross elongation and distortion of the cervix and uterine body (**a**), cobblestone endometrial hyperplasia (**d**) and obstructed left tube (**c**).

C, uterosalpingogram, right posterior oblique projection: Showing marked extrinsic distortion of the uterine cavity.

D, uterosalpingogram, left posterior oblique projection: Confirming the extrinsic deformity of the uterine cavity by fibroid tumor.

A 22-year-old married nulliparous woman complained of some menorrhagia for four months and intermenstrual bleeding for two months. An enlarged uterus was palpable on pelvic examination; a pregnancy test was negative. The radiologic studies strongly supported the diagnosis of uterine fibroid tumor. Plans for preoperative dilatation and curettage were canceled after the uterosalpingogram showed conspicuous distortion of the cervical canal. A 9 cm diffuse fibroid tumor of the uterus and cystic right ovary required hysterectomy and right salpingo-oophorectomy.

Figure 14 from Stevens, G. M., *et al.:* M. Radiog. & Photog. 42:82, 1966.

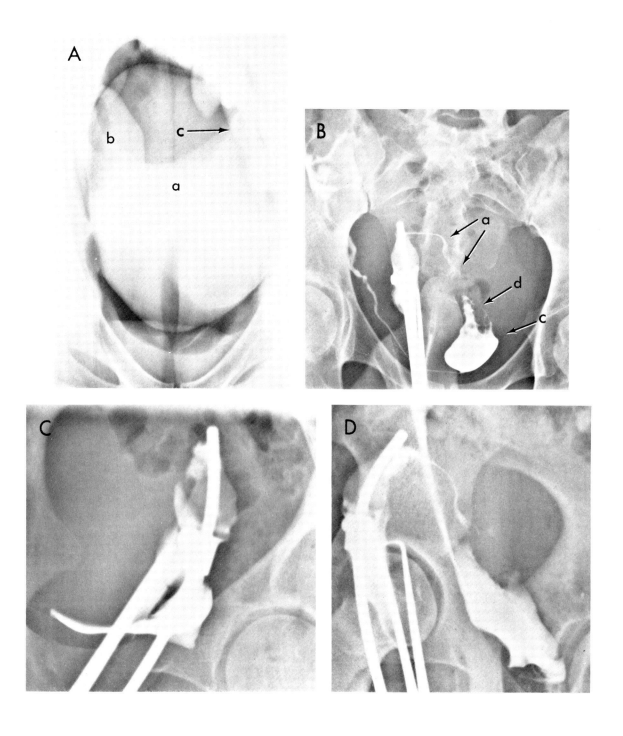

Figure 14 · Large Fibroid in Young Woman / 43

Figure 15.—Uterine fibroids: pelvic pneumography.

A, posteroanterior projection: Revealing a multinodular uterine outline, indicative of multiple small intramural fibroids, and bilateral cystic enlargement of the ovaries (2 × normal size).

B, right anterior oblique projection: Showing irregular uterine outline (**a**) and cystic left ovary (**b**). The right ovary (**c**) is partially obscured by the uterus.

A 41-year-old multiparous woman had regular menses and menorrhagia. Recent cytologic studies suggested carcinoma of the cervix. Following pelvic pneumography she had a hysterectomy, and bilateral ovarian wedge biopsy specimens were obtained. Multiple small uterine myomas, in situ carcinoma of the cervix and bilateral ovarian follicular cysts were found.

C, posteroanterior projection: Demonstrating enlarged uterus due to multiple, moderate-size fibroids (**a**), slightly enlarged right ovary (**arrows**) and normal left ovary (**b**).

D, lateral projection: Showing the irregular uterine outline due to fibroids (**arrows**).

This 44-year-old para 6 woman had regular menses. Routine pelvic examination disclosed uterine fibroids and a suspected right ovarian mass. At surgery, fibroids were found and a slightly cystic right ovary, but no tumor.

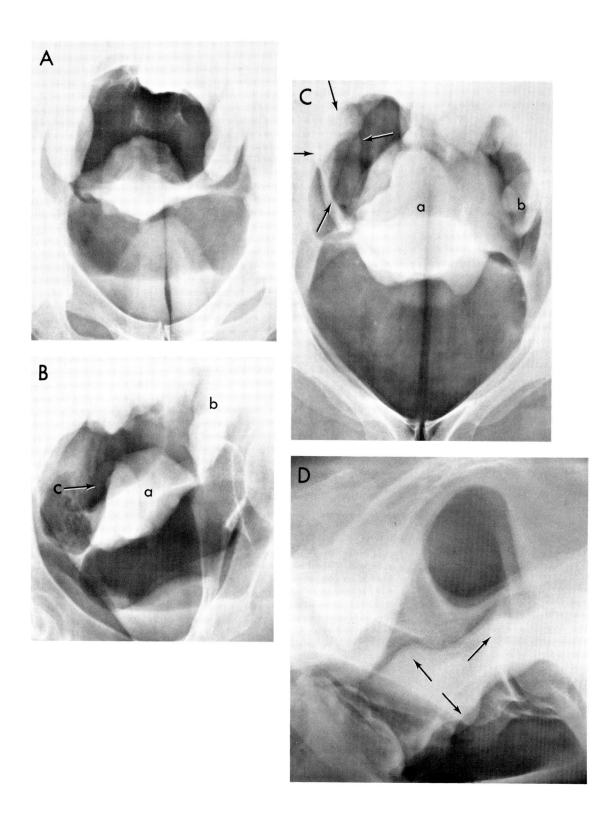

Figure 15 · Fibroids: Pelvic Pneumography / 45

Figure 16.—Uterine fibroids: pelvic pneumography (posteroanterior projections).

A, Large subserous fibroid (**a**) is attached to the right anterior aspect of the uterus (**b**). The right ovary (**c**) is slightly enlarged, the left ovary (**d**) normal.

A multiparous woman, age 34, had a history of urinary frequency, irregular menses, dysmenorrhea and occasional menorrhagia. The gynecologist could not confidently distinguish between a uterine fibroid and an attached ovarian neoplasm to explain the palpable mass.

B, Numerous subserosal and intramural fibroids (**arrows**) distort and enlarge the uterine outline. Pneumatized colon (**x**). The ovaries are obscured by fibroids.

A woman of 46 had had occasional right lower quadrant pain with the menses. Pelvic examination on three occasions by two internists was negative. Presence of multiple uterine fibroids seen on the pneumogram was confirmed during gallbladder surgery.

C, There is generalized uterine enlargement due to multiple intramural fibroids, one of which (**a**) is calcified. Ovaries (**arrows**) are normal.

A gravida II patient of 40 was found on routine physical examination to have a pelvic mass of uncertain origin. Pelvic pneumography was done for clarification. Surgery confirmed the diagnosis of fibroids.

D, Large fibroid (**a**) is attached to the posterior right aspect of the uterus (**b**). The ovaries are obscured.

A para 5 patient, age 39, had erosion of the cervix and a moderate cystocele and rectocele. The uterus seemed enlarged, but physical examination was difficult because of heavy musculature and obesity. After pelvic pneumography, subtotal hysterectomy and pelvic floor repair were done. An 8 cm fibroid was attached to the posterior right aspect of the uterus.

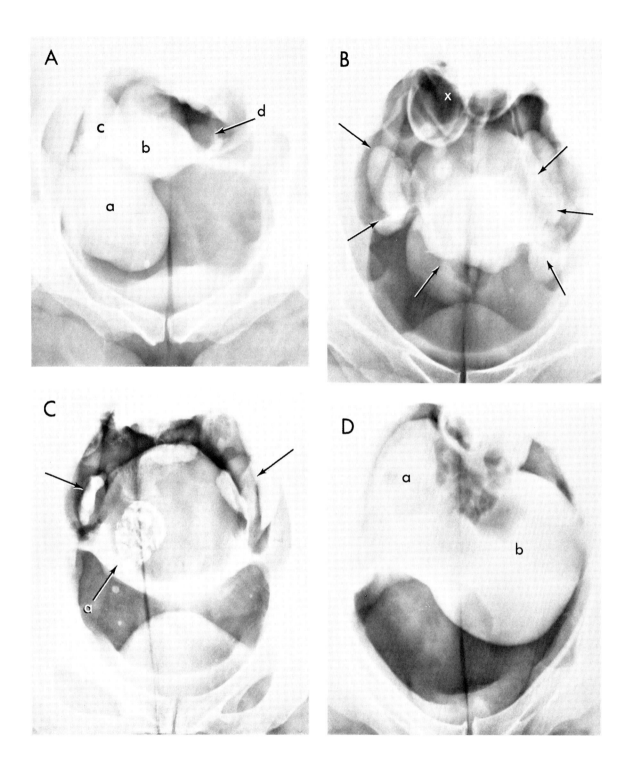

Figure 16 · Fibroids: Pelvic Pneumography / 47

Figure 17.—Uterine fibroids: pelvic pneumography.

A, posteroanterior projection: Showing marked anteroposterior enlargement of the uterine fundus (**a**) due to intramural and small subserosal fibroids (**arrows**). Right ovary (**b**). Left ovary not seen.

B, right anterior oblique projection: Demonstrating the fibroid uterus (**a**) and subserosal fibroid (**arrow**).

A single, gravida 0 woman of 28 had normal menses except for recent pre- and postmenstrual spotting. The uterus was firm and enlarged to twice normal size. A cyst of the right ovary was suspected. Cytologic examination was normal. Pelvic pneumography confirmed uterine enlargement consistent with uterine fibroids. Surgery was not performed because of the patient's age and desire for eventual maternity.

C, posteroanterior projection: Demonstrating marked uterine enlargement (**arrows**) due to fibroids, some of which contain calcifications (**x**). The ovaries are obscured by the uterus. Pedunculated fibroid (**c**).

D, right anterior oblique projection: Showing fibroid enlargement of the uterus (**arrows**), calcification in the fibroid in the right posterior aspect of the uterus (**x**) and a pedunculated fibroid (**c**).

During an annual physical examination a 41-year-old unmarried virginal woman was found to have a firm pelvic mass. The ovaries could not be palpated. The mass was assumed to be due to uterine fibroids; a pelvic pneumogram was ordered for confirmation. Hysterectomy and left oophorectomy were performed, with removal of multiple uterine fibroids (up to 7 cm diameter) and a corpus luteum cyst.

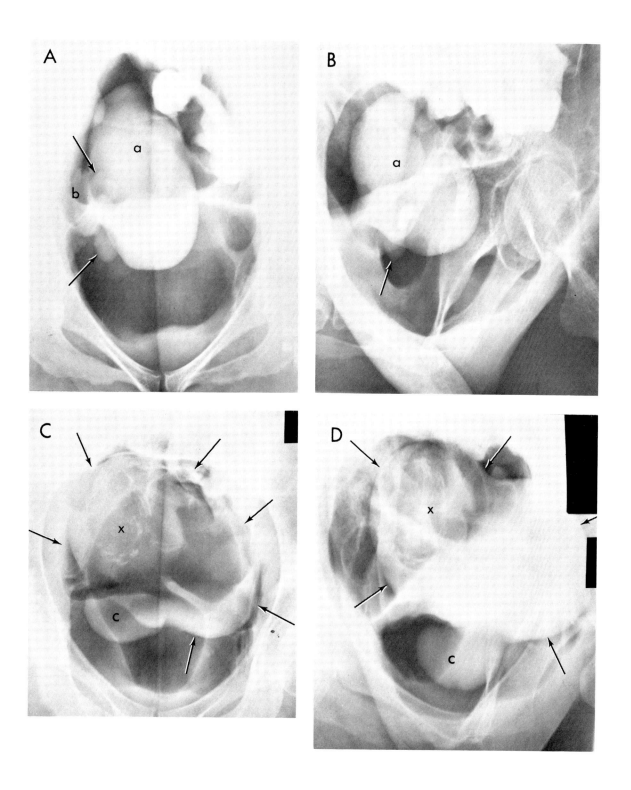

Figure 17 · Fibroids: Pelvic Pneumography / 49

Figure 18.—Large fibroid uterus: pelvic pneumography.

A, posteroanterior view: Showing moderate uterine enlargement due to multiple intrauterine fibroids (**a**) and a 7 cm intraligamentous fibroid (**b**) in the right broad ligament. The right ovary is not seen. The left ovary seems slightly enlarged (**c**).

B, right anterior oblique projection: An intraligamentous fibroid (**b**) causing widening of the right broad ligament (**d**). Adhesions (**e**); left ovary (**c**).

C, left anterior oblique projection: Showing slightly cystic right ovary (**arrows**).

A 42-year-old gravida I para 0 patient described vaginal spotting for three or four days following cessation of menstruation during the last four periods. The uterus was considerably enlarged on palpation and had grown since the previous year's examination. A firm large mass was attached to the right side of the uterus. Because of the possibility of an ovarian tumor, pelvic pneumography was ordered. Surgery revealed a large intraligamentous fibroid on the right and multiple small intramural fibroids. The right ovary was slightly enlarged due to cystic change; the left one was normal.

Comment: Both ovaries are somewhat magnified in the films owing to their posterior displacement due to uterine enlargement.

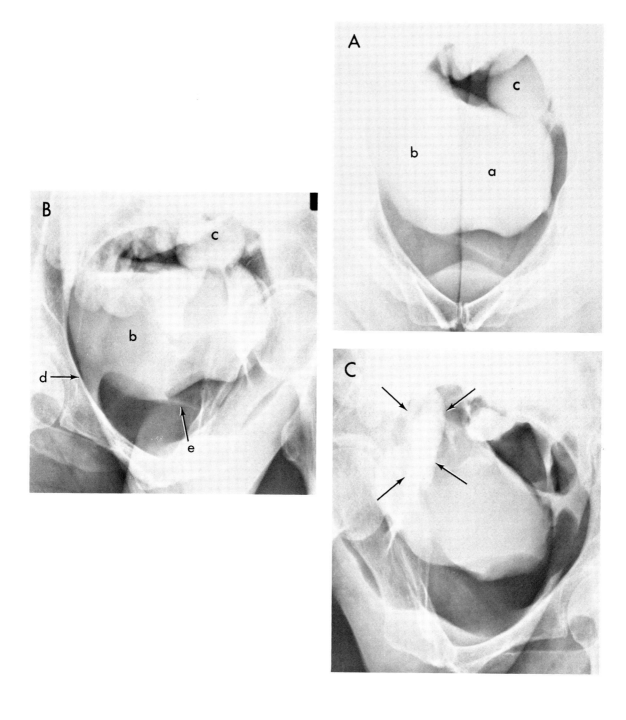

Figure 18 · Fibroids: Pelvic Pneumography / 51

Figure 19.—Multiple uterine fibroids.

A, anteroposterior view: Showing a sausage-shaped peripherally calcified mass in the right pelvis.

B, pelvic pneumogram, posteroanterior projection: Demonstrating distortion and enlargement of the uterus (**a**) and a pedunculated peripherally calcified uterine fibroid (**b**).

C, uterosalpingogram, anteroposterior view: Revealing marked deformity of the uterine cavity by intramural fibroids.

D, uterosalpingogram, left posterior oblique projection: Showing uterine cavity distortion.

A 34-year-old gravida I woman had had menometrorrhagia for six or seven months. Secondary infertility had persisted for five years following four spontaneous abortions. The uterus was enlarged to three or four times normal size and was irregular in outline, with several attached subserous fibroids. Dilatation and curettage were performed. The sensation of uterine fibroids was noted on curettage. Similar symptoms, followed by dilatation and curettage, occurred three and five years later.

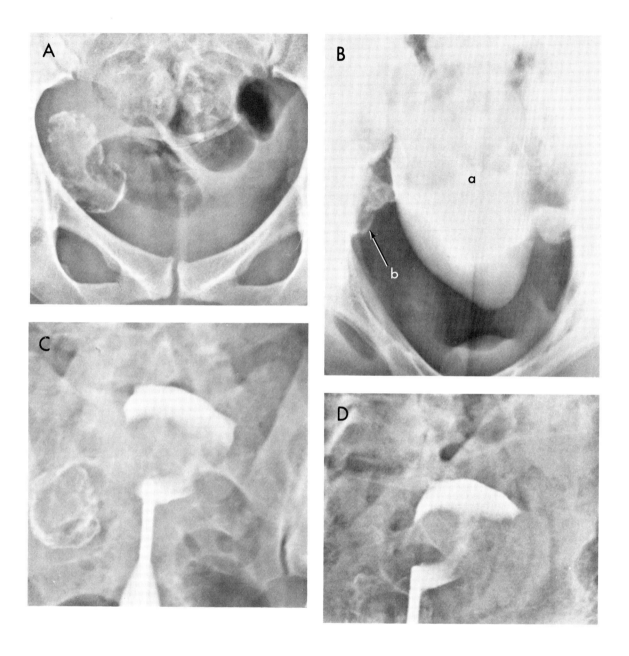

Figure 19 · Multiple Fibroids / 53

Figure 20.—Uterine fibroids: pelvic pneumography.

A, posteroanterior projection: Showing marked uterine enlargement (**a**). The left ovary (**b**) is normal; the right ovary is not seen.

B, right anterior oblique view: Separating the outline of the uterine mass (**a**), believed due to fibroids, and the right ovary (**c**).

C, lateral prone projection: Illustrating the uterine fibroid mass.

A 44-year-old woman with a history of occasional menorrhagia came for a periodic physical examination. Uterine fibroids had been diagnosed 10 years before. Now a mass filled the pelvis, precluding examination of the adnexa. Concern was raised about the mass being of ovarian origin. Pelvic pneumography was requested to clarify this question since the patient had declined surgery.

Comment: A large mass filling the pelvis is considered by some to be a contraindication for pelvic pneumography (on the basis that it is useless). Exceptions to this are fairly common (as in this case), though diagnosis is often undeniably difficult and sometimes impossible in these circumstances.

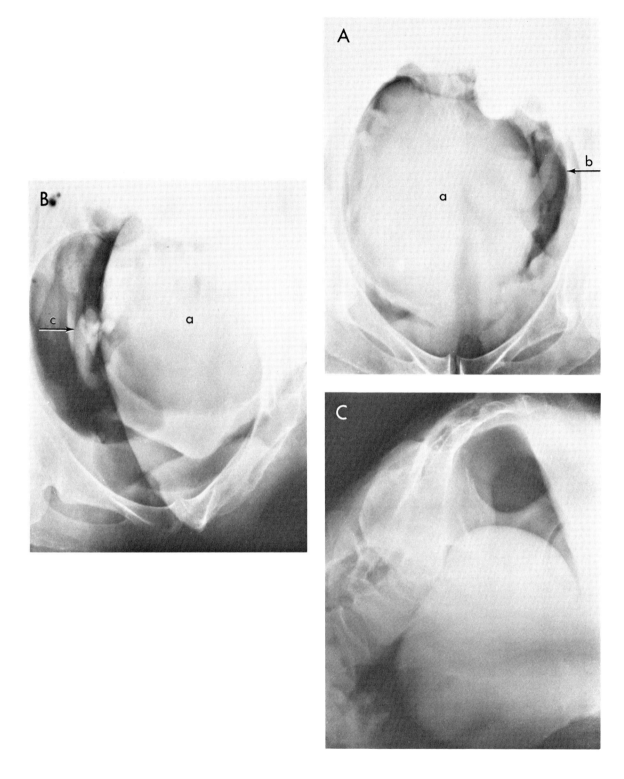

Figure 20 · Fibroids: Pelvic Pneumography / 55

Figure 21.—Uterine fibroids: pelvic pneumography.

A, posteroanterior view: Showing marked lobular enlargement of the uterus due to fibroids (**a**), the uterine isthmus (**b**) displaced to the right, and normal left ovary (**c**).

B, left anterior oblique projection: Demonstrating fibroid enlargement of the uterus (**a**), and the right ovary (**d**).

A gravida 0 patient, age 38, had an enlarging firm mass in the left adnexa. First diagnosed four years previously, it was believed to be a pedunculated fibroid, but because the gynecologist feared that the mass arose from the left ovary, pelvic pneumography was ordered. At surgery a 9 cm fibroma of the uterus was removed, as well as a moderate-size corpus luteum cyst from the right ovary.

C, posteroanterior projection: Showing lobular enlargement of the uterine fundus due to fibroids (**a**), the ovaries (**c**) and a small paraovarian cyst (**e**).

D, slight right anterior oblique projection: Showing the lobular fibroid uterus (**a**). Ovarian outlines are now not easily distinguished from the bowel.

A para 2 woman of 48 complained of intermenstrual pain for 2½ years. Pelvic examination was unsatisfactory. The fundus was believed to be at the upper limit of normal size and the left adnexa thickened. Hysterectomy disclosed multiple intramural fibroids from 3–5 cm in size.

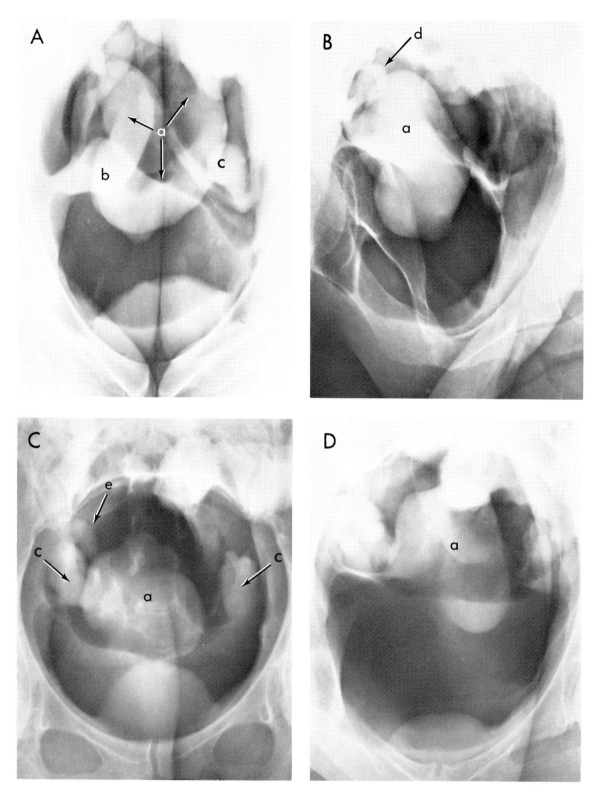

Figure 21 · Fibroids: Pelvic Pneumography / 57

Figure 22.—Intraligamentous fibroid tumor; subserous uterine fibroid: pelvic pneumograms.

A, posteroanterior projection: Showing a large left adnexal mass (**a**) which widens the broad ligament and extends to the left pelvic wall. (Note the normal right broad ligament (**b**) for comparison.) Uterus (**c**); right ovary (**d**).

B, left anterior oblique view: Better illustrating the intraligamentous position of the lobular fibroid tumor (**a**). Note widening of the left broad ligament (between **arrows**). Uterus (**c**); right ovary (**d**).

A patient, age 40, noted needlelike pelvic discomfort while reclining and suspected recurrence of endometriosis. Sixteen years before she had had a left oophorectomy for an endometrioma and removal of small uterine fibroids. No abnormality was noted on pelvic examination four months previously, but now a mass in the left adnexa was questionably palpable. At surgery an intraligamentous fibroid tumor was found on the left.

C, posteroanterior projection: Showing a small pedunculated subserous fibroid arising from the posterior right side of the uterus (**e**), and the uterus eccentrically positioned toward the patient's left (**f**). Right ovary (**d**); left ovary obscured; sigmoid colon (**x**).

D, right anterior oblique projection: Separating the uterine fibroid (**e**) from the sigmoid (**x**). Uterus (**c**); right ovary (**d**); left ovary (**g**).

A 29-year-old woman had a premarital examination, at which time a pelvic mass was suspected. Because its origin was not clear, pelvic pneumography was ordered.

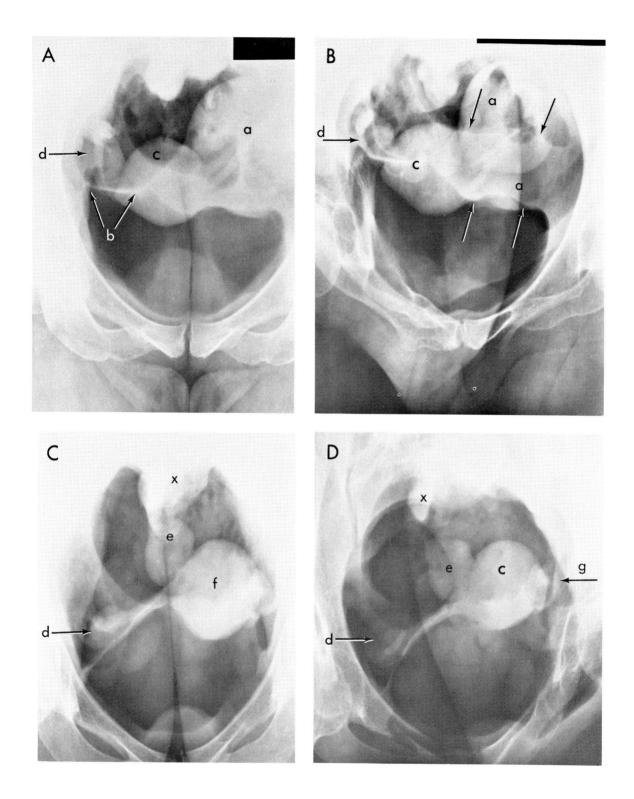

Figure 22 · Intraligamentous & Subserous Fibroids / 59

Figure 23.—Lithopedion simulating uterine fibroid with small bowel obstruction.

A, anteroposterior supine exposure: Showing calcified mass simulating a uterine fibroid, proved to be skeletal residue of a nonviable ectopic pregnancy, with mechanical obstruction of the ileum due to an adhesive band.

B, left lateral decubitus position: Note fluid levels and position of calcified mass (**x**).

C, radiograph of specimen, clearly demonstrating the fetal skeleton.

A 40-year-old patient entered the hospital complaining of cramping abdominal pain for six days. No flatus or fecal material had been passed during this interval. An adhesive band passed from the fetal remnant of the ectopic pregnancy to obstruct the ileum.

Figure 23, courtesy of Dr. R. H. Chamberlain, University of Pennsylvania, Philadelphia.

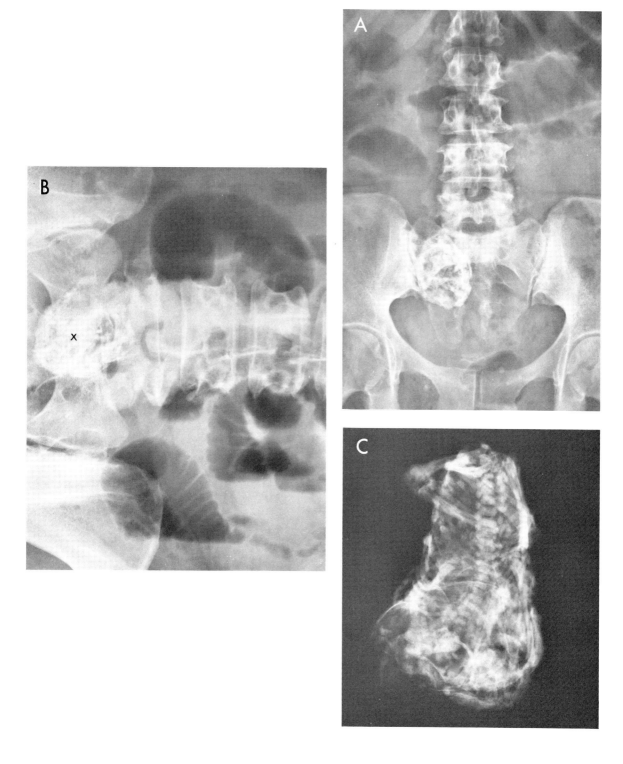

Figure 23 · Lithopedion Simulating Fibroid / 61

Figure 24.—Uterine fibroids in pregnancy.

A, anteroposterior projection: Showing lobular enlargement (**a**) of normal pregnant uterine outline. Note fetal skeletal parts in uterus (**x**).

A primigravida, age 31, was hospitalized in the sixth month with cramping left lower quadrant pain. There was slight diarrhea but no nausea or vomiting. It was known from early pregnancy that a small fibroid was present on the left side of the uterus. In a few hours symptoms had progressed so that surgery was required. A 15 × 12 × 10 cm multilobular degenerating cystic fibroid was removed from the anterior left surface of the uterus, and a 3 × 5 cm fibroid from the uterine dome. At term a normal infant was delivered by cesarean section.

B, anteroposterior view: Curvilinear calcification in the periphery of a uterine fibroid in the right upper abdomen (**arrow**) simulates a second fetal head.

A woman, 25, in the third trimester, had an abdominal radiograph made to determine fetal position. The calcification seen in **B** was intially misinterpreted as a second fetal skull, presumably a dead twin associated with a normal pregnancy.

B, courtesy of Dr. A. K. Briney, Whittier, Calif.

C, anteroposterior view: A smooth-bordered mass (**b**) extends into the left midabdomen from a 3-month pregnant uterus.

A gravida I, para 0 patient, age 32, had first cramping, then constant pain in the left lower quadrant. Pain in the left pelvis was present on walking, and a tender mass in this area was noted on palpation. The mass was not present on examination four days before. A 10 × 8 × 8 cm hemorrhagic degenerating fibroid was removed from the left cornual area of the uterus. She aborted a week later.

Comment: Uterine myomas generally enlarge during pregnancy, then regress. Degeneration of the myoma during this period of rapid growth is not unusual.

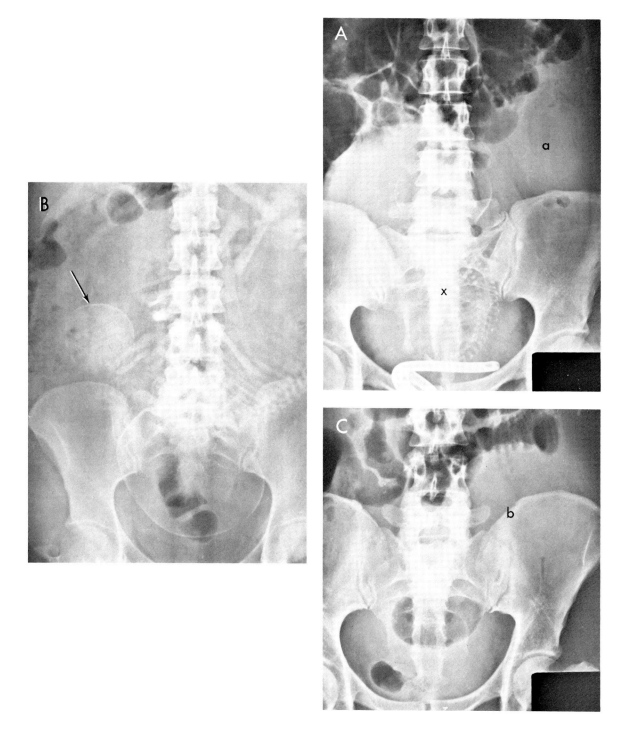

Figure 24 · Fibroids in Pregnancy / 63

Figure 25.—Uterine fibroid: pelvic arteriograms (anteroposterior views).

A, early arterial phase: **4,** uterine artery; **9,** superior rectal artery; **10,** right ovarian artery.

B, midarterial phase: **4,** uterine artery; **9,** superior rectal artery; **10,** right ovarian artery. **a,** uterine arteries deflected to left indicating uterine displacement; **b,** early opacification of arteries to large right uterine fibroid.

(*Continued* on page 66.)

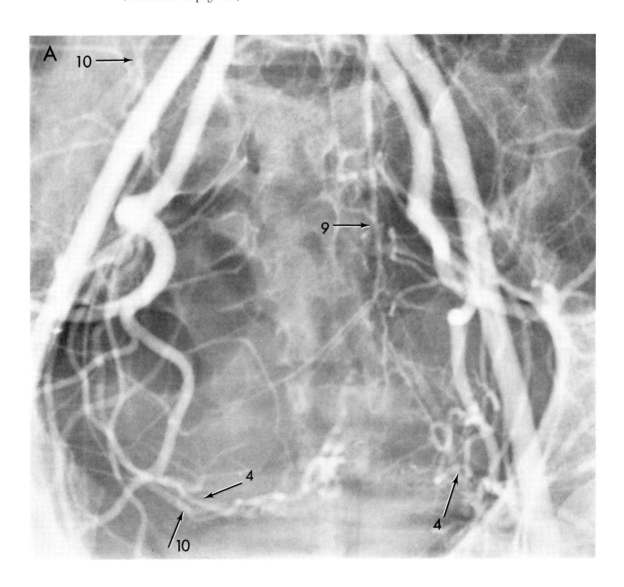

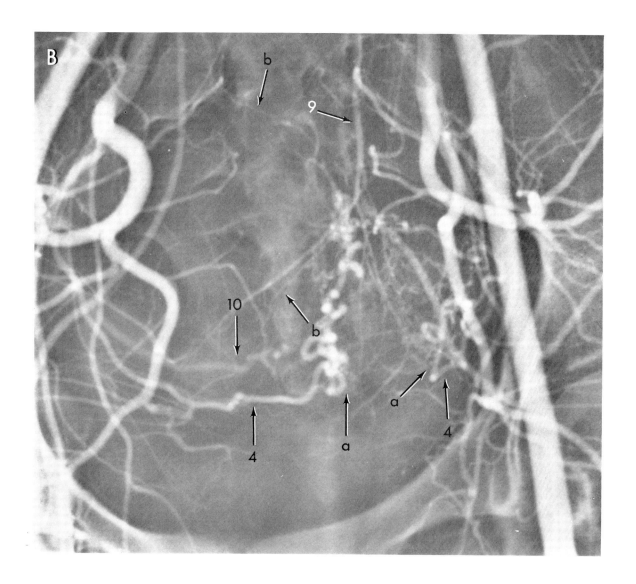

Figure 25 · Fibroids: Pelvic Arteriography / 65

Figure 25 (cont.).—Uterine fibroid: pelvic arteriograms.

C, late arterial phase: Uterus, now well vascularized (**a**), is deflected to left. Arched and stretched tributaries (**c**) from the right uterine artery extend to the relatively avascular right uterine fibroid.

A woman, age 44, had a one month history of metrorrhagia and a mass the size of a billiard ball to the right of the uterus. A slightly pedunculated subserous uterine fibroid was found.

Comment: This fibroid is somewhat less vascular than some are.

Figure 25, courtesy of Drs. C. Rådberg and I. Wickbom, Gothenberg, Sweden.

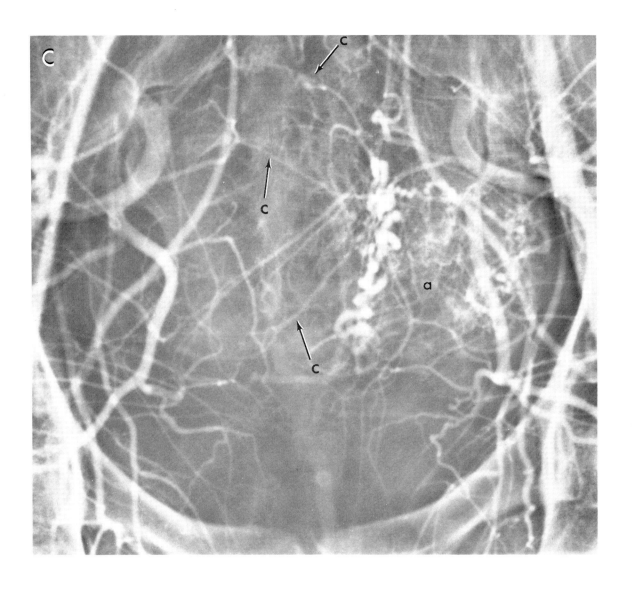

Figure 25 · Fibroids: Pelvic Arteriography / 67

Figure 26.—Large uterine fibroid: pelvic arteriograms (anteroposterior views).

A, early arterial phase: Showing enlarged uterine arteries (**4**) widely separated by large central fibroid tumors. At least two are present, as seen by the separate arcuate contours (**a** and **b**) within the mass. Large corkscrew type vessels run within the substance of the fibroid, and capsular vessels circumscribe its periphery.

B, late arterial phase: delineating innumerable tiny tumor vessels within the highly vascularized large uterine fibroid (**arrows**).

The patient, age 61, was seen because of marked uterine enlargement.

Figure 26, courtesy of Drs. C. Rådberg and I. Wickbom, Gothenberg, Sweden.

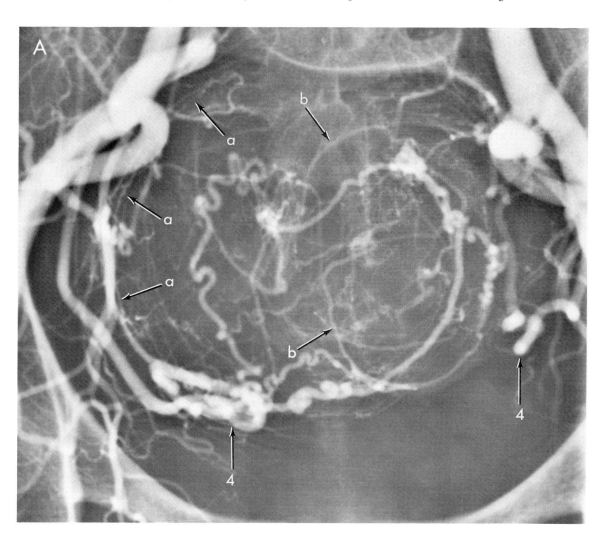

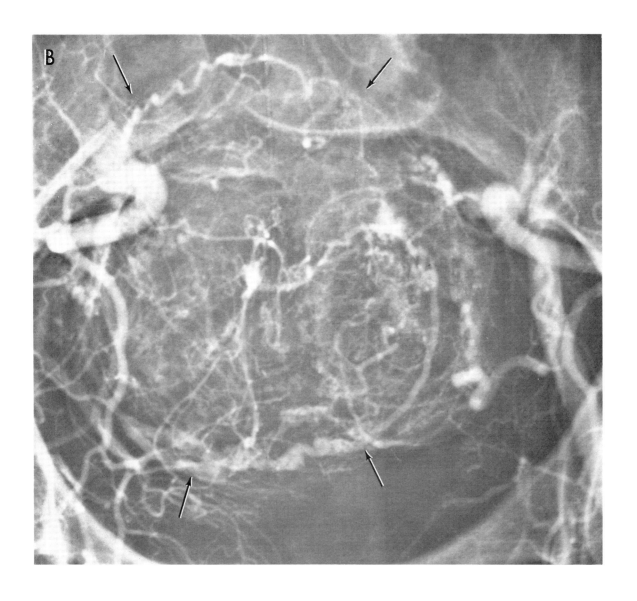

Figure 26 · Fibroid: Pelvic Arteriography / 69

Figure 27.—Uterine fibroid: pelvic arteriograms (anteroposterior views).

A, arterial phase: Uterine arteries (**4**); many large arched and stretched tributaries from the left uterine artery (**a**). The uterus is deflected to the right, as indicated by the normal intramural branches of the right uterine artery (**b**).

B, arterial-venous phase: The size and contour of the uterine fibroid can now be more distinctly seen (**arrows**). Uterine body (**open arrows**).

A woman, age 26, had experienced metrorrhagia for three months and had acute salpingitis two months before admission. An initially tender mass inseparable from the left side of the uterus grew smaller, firm and nontender. A uterine fibroid was found at surgery.

Figure 27, courtesy of Drs. C. Rådberg and I. Wickbom, Gothenberg, Sweden.

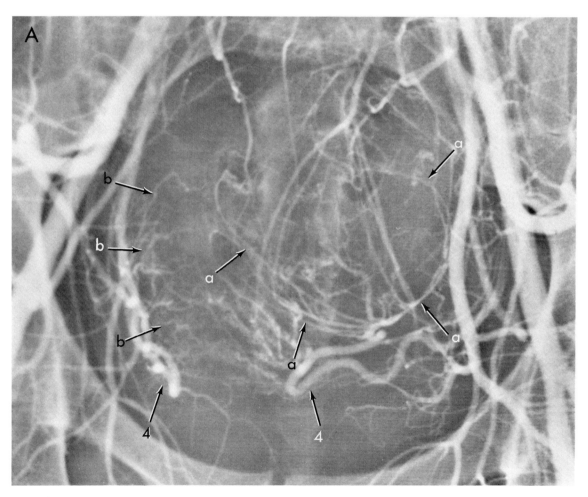

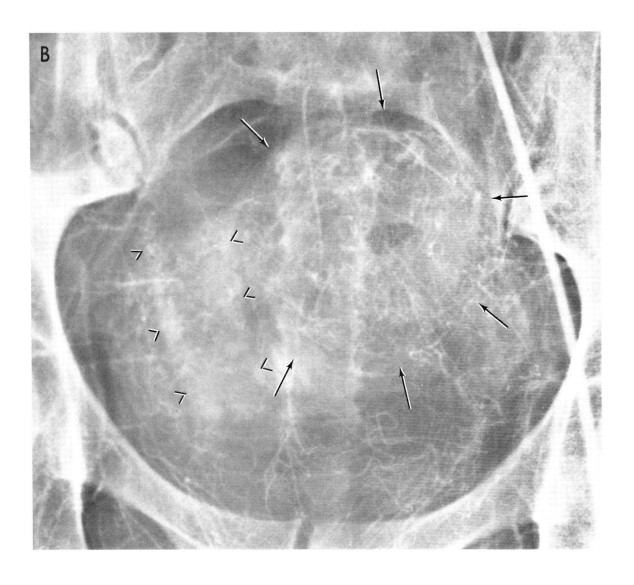

Figure 27 · Fibroids: Pelvic Arteriography / 71

Figure 28.—Endometrial polyps: uterosalpingograms.

A, anteroposterior view, after instillation of only 2 cc of water-soluble contrast medium: Showing two small endometrial polyps (**arrows**) and the uterus situated to the left of the midline.

B, anteroposterior view after instillation of 6 cc: The polyps are now nearly obscured (**arrows**).

C, left posterior oblique projection: Polyps are barely seen. The tubes are patent bilaterally.

A woman, age 25, had not conceived during two years of marriage despite normal ovulation and menstruation, normal physical examination and normal Rubin's test.

Comment: The importance of fractional filling under fluoroscopic guidance is emphasized in this case. Contrast which is either too radiopaque or too voluminous may obscure intracavity abnormalities.

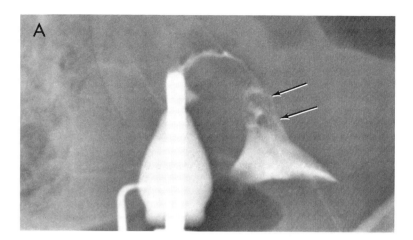

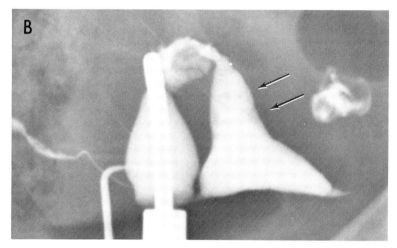

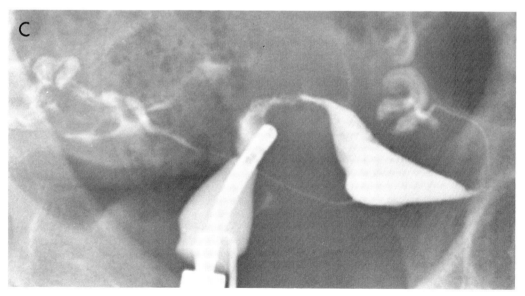

Figure 28 · Endometrial Polyps / 73

Hysterography in Cancer of the Uterus

by OLOF NORMAN, M.D.*

HYSTEROSALPINGOGRAPHY HAS BEEN primarily used in the investigation of female sterility, but its value in the detection and evaluation of uterine carcinoma should not be overlooked. Hitherto the method has been used by only a few workers for this purpose, Béclère being the first to use hysterography routinely in the evaluation of metrorrhagia. The roentgen diagnostic department and the gynecological section of the radium therapy department at the University of Lund Hospital have collaborated since 1946 in routinely using this technique in the study of cancer of the uterus, mainly of the corpus.[5] During this time 3000 examinations on approximately 1800 patients have been conducted.

TECHNIQUE.—A standard hysterosalpingography technique is utilized; however, a selection of cones of various sizes should be available to assure a good fit with the cervix. The nozzle of the cannula should project only a few millimeters beyond the cone, this being necessary not only to minimize the risk of perforation but also to allow visualization of any changes in the cervix.

Iodized oil is not suitable for this type of examination. It does not bring out the finer details of the outline of the tumor nor does it mix with the secretion often present in cancer. The risk of vascular embolization also represents a disadvantage of oily contrast. For 15 years we have used Perjodal-H-Viscous, a diiodinated pyridon to which dextran has been added as a thickener.

The examination must be carried out under fluoroscopic control. This direct visualization permits the examiner to follow the passage of the contrast medium into the uterine cavity and to take films with optimal filling in the necessary positions.

THEORETICAL HAZARDS.—The main reason hysterography is not used more widely in the investigation of cancer is that many authors have exaggerated the possible risks attending the method. Our experience from more than 3000 cancer examinations justifies the following statements.

---

* Roentgen Diagnostic Department, University Hospital, Lund, Sweden.
[5] Norman, O.: Hysterography in cancer of the corpus of the uterus, Acta radiol., Supp. 79, p. 255, 1950; Seminars Roentgenol. 4:244, 1969.

A certain risk of instrumental injury attends hysterography just as it does instrumental palpation and curettage. The frequency of mechanical injury is, however, the same in cancer patients as in patients without malignancy.

The possibility of cancer dissemination by hysterography is often used as an argument against employment of the method. In our series a follow-up study has been made by my associate John-Erik Johnson, who found no evidence to confirm this theoretical hazard.

Since local infection fairly commonly accompanies cancer of the uterus, a careful study has been made to assess the risk of infection being spread by hysterography. This risk has proved to be no greater than that experienced in routine hysterosalpingography.

RELIABILITY.—The value of hysterography for the diagnosis of uterine cancer is established by the fact that during 22 years in which 1800 uterine cancer patients were examined, tumor was missed in only one case. In approximately 10% of these patients the first evidence of malignancy was established by hysterography within a few months of one or more negative curettages. Half of these tumors were large.

Certain benign endometrial processes may simulate carcinoma and lead to occasional false positive diagnosis. Among the localized expansive processes which may simulate carcinoma are sarcoma, myoma, polyps, pregnancy, hydatidiform mole and placental remnants. Endometrial hyperplasia and endometritis are characteristically diffuse and involve the entire endometrium, while carcinoma tends to be localized in most patients.

INDICATIONS.—Despite our good results, hysterography is not indicated in all cases. Its most useful application falls in the following three categories: (1) patients suspected of having carcinoma in whom curettage is negative; (2) assistance in treatment planning by providing evidence of location, size and extent of the tumor, and (3) assessment of the effectiveness of radiation therapy during or following treatment.

NOTE: Figures 29–38 were generously furnished by Dr. Norman.—G.M.S.

Figure 29.—Carcinomas of the endometrium, highly differentiated and poorly differentiated types: hysterograms.

A, anteroposterior view: Showing the uterus to be slightly enlarged and, with the exception of the lower part of the body, to be entirely filled with cancer having a very irregular outline. This appearance is typical of a highly differentiated tumor.

The patient, age 60, was examined because of postmenopausal bleeding.

B, anteroposterior view (another patient): Showing the uterus filled and expanded by a smoothly outlined, well-demarcated tumor growing from the left wall of the uterus. Cancer of this appearance is generally poorly differentiated.

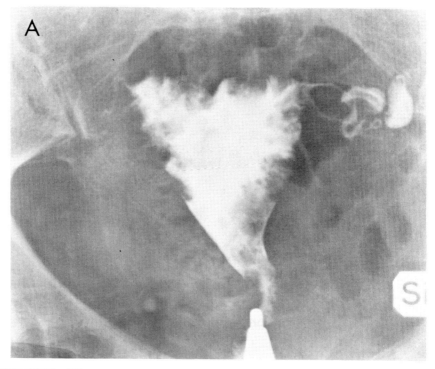

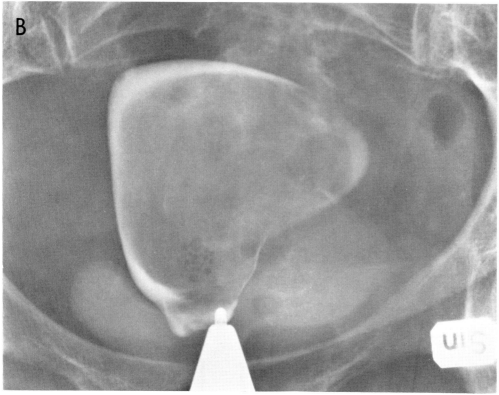

Figure 29 · Endometrial Carcinomas / 77

Figure 30.—Carcinomas of the endometrium: hysterograms.

A, anteroposterior projection: delineating a ragged, fairly exophytic tumor in the left uterine wall. Thanks to the contrast medium in the abdomen, the uterine surface is outlined, thereby allowing estimation of the thickness of the uterine wall; such an estimate cannot be obtained routinely.

Comment: After the menopause, the tubes are closed in about 50% of women, although they were not in this patient.

B, anteroposterior view (of another patient): Showing the greater part of the uterine wall occupied by irregular changes which could represent hyperplasia or possibly highly differentiated cancer. Because hyperplasia usually involves the entire endometrium and since the left part of the uterus is free from changes, the diagnosis was probable cancer. Initial biopsy, however, showed no evidence of tumor.

The 37-year-old patient was examined because of irregular bleeding. Because of the roentgen diagnosis, biopsy studies were repeated one month and three months later, giving first a diagnosis of hyperplasia and finally of carcinoma.

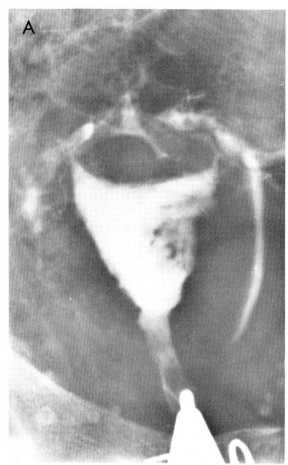

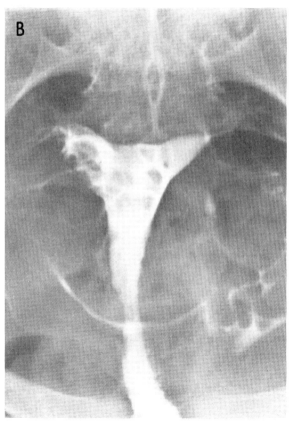

Figure 30 · Endometrial Carcinomas / 79

Figure 31.—Uterine carcinoma with myoma: hysterogram.

Anteroposterior projection: Revealing a large myoma (**a**) almost occluding the cervix, and cancer (**b**) in the left upper part of the body.

This menopausal patient was examined because of bleeding. Curettage gave negative results. Because of the findings on palpation a cervical cancer was suspected and hysterography ordered. Apparently the myoma had prevented the curet from passing into the uterine cavity.

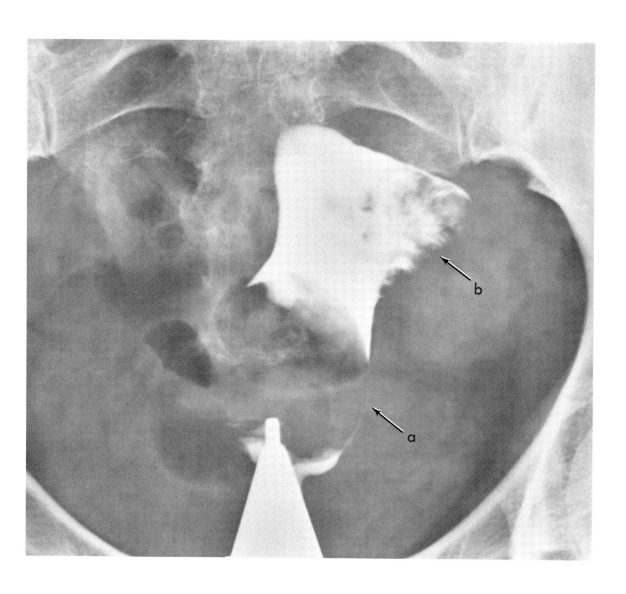

Figure 31 · Uterine Carcinoma with Myoma / 81

Figure 32.—Uterine carcinomas: hysterograms.

A, anteroposterior view: Showing the enlarged uterus and in the left wall a polypoid exophytic growth from which a low ridgelike extension (**arrows**) continues down into the cervix.

In this patient, curettage yielded ample tissue from the cervix and a diagnosis of adenocarcinoma was made, but only a small area of the anterior wall of the corpus could be curetted and no tumor tissue was obtained. The roentgen picture, which corresponded in every respect with the surgical specimen, shows how the expansive corpus tumor bulges over the internal os, thereby allowing only a small range of movement of the curet in an attempt to remove tissue from the corpus.

Comment: Hysterography can be helpful in distinguishing the cervical from the uterine fundus origin of a tumor, as in this case, in which fractional curettage failed to demonstrate the uterine origin of the carcinoma with extension into the cervix.

B, anteroposterior projection: Revealing a fairly large bulging tumor in the right lower part of the uterine body.

In this 75-year-old woman, a diagnosis of cervical cancer was based on curet palpation and fractional curettage. No cancer tissue was obtained from the uterine body. The tumor was apparently inaccessible to instruments passing up through the cervix.

Comment: Hysterography has proved to be definitely superior to instrumental exploration in showing the spread of the tumor.

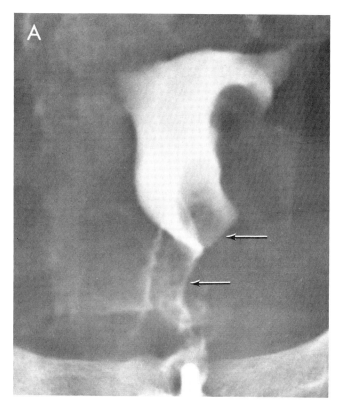

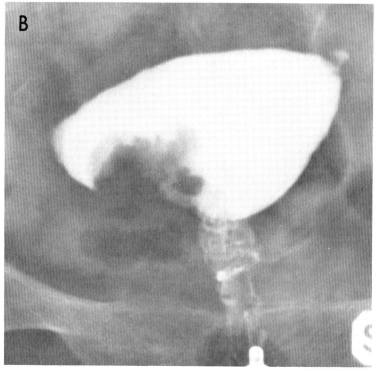

Figure 32 · Uterine Carcinoma Involving Cervix / 83

Figure 33.—Uterine carcinoma with pyometra: hysterogram.

Anteroposterior projection: Showing the uterus transformed into a large sac with multiple mural changes. This picture has proved to be characteristic of pyometra complicating endometrial carcinoma.

This patient, age 72, had a history of vaginal discharge and bleeding for 18 months.

Comment: Hysterography can be of great help in planning the treatment. Knowledge of the uterine topography is important in deciding on the size and number of radium capsules when a packing technique is used.

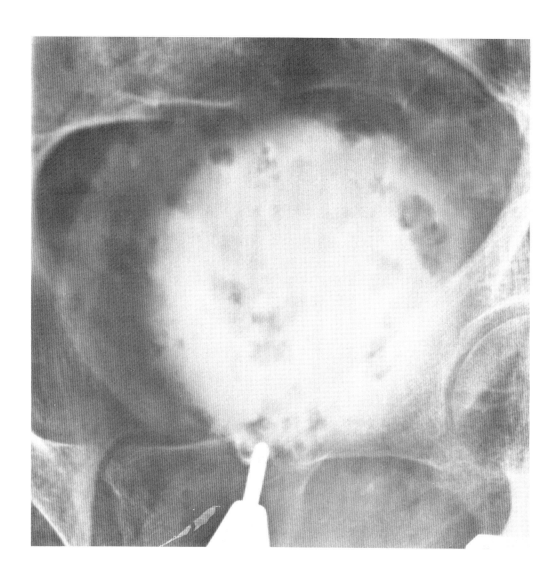

Figure 33 · Uterine Carcinoma with Pyometra / 85

Figure 34.—Uterine carcinoma, undetected by curettage.

Hysterography series, demonstrating the importance of fluoroscopic control.

A, anteroposterior view: Showing the uterus to be flexed.

B, right posterior oblique view: Showing the uterus anteflexed. Neither **A** nor **B** reveals pathologic changes.

C, left posterior oblique view with optimal angulation under fluoroscopic control: Disclosing a small, well-demarcated carcinoma in the left uterine horn (**arrows**).

The patient, aged 68, after one month's postmenopausal bleeding submitted to curettage by a specialist. No tumor was instrumentally palpable, and microscopic examination of curetted tissues showed nothing pathologic. As the bleeding persisted, hysterography was performed and the tumor located. Repeat curettage was carried out the following day under guidance of the hysterogram. The tumor was palpated but no tissue could be removed despite repeated attempts. At operation on the following day a circumscribed, extremely firm cancer was found in the left horn.

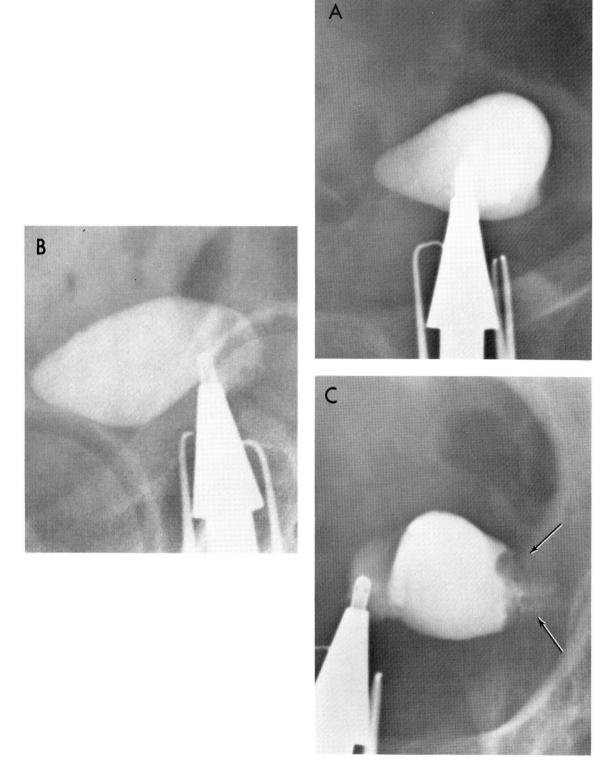

Figure 34 · Uterine Carcinoma / 87

Figure 35.—Endometrial carcinoma in right horn of a bicornuate uterus: hysterogram.

Left posterior oblique view: Delineating cancer in one horn of a bicornuate uterus.

Comment: This condition often escapes diagnosis by curettage, as in this case. During instrumental exploration, the normal horn may be entered, a normal uterine cavity depth noted and no suspicion of anatomic variation entertained. Eleven such cases have been encountered at the University of Lund.

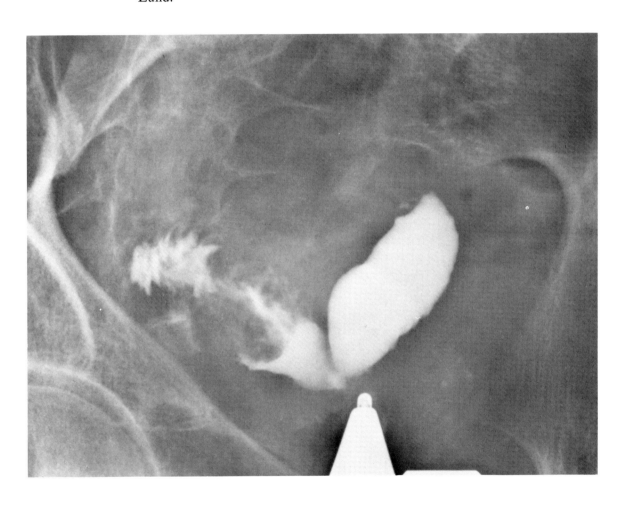

Figure 36.—Fungating endometrial carcinoma, undetected by curettage: hysterogram.

Left posterior oblique projections: Showing the body of the uterus almost filled with cancer, and the uterus markedly flexed, which probably accounts for failure of curettage to detect the tumor.

Hysterography was performed in this patient of 63 because of persistent bleeding, the cause of which was obscure after two negative curettements. Hysterography is an excellent method for discovering pathologic changes in the uterus when anatomic variations make curettage difficult.

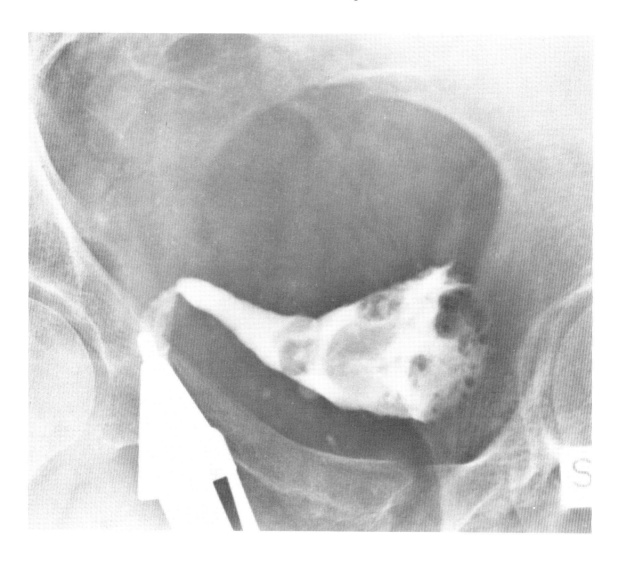

Figure 36 · Fungating Endometrial Carcinoma / 89

Figure 37.—Uterine carcinoma: control hysterograms to follow response to therapy.

A, slightly left posterior oblique projection, prior to treatment: Revealing a highly organized cancer in the left part of the uterine body.

B, anteroposterior view, during treatment: demonstrating diminution of the tumor.

C, slightly right posterior oblique projection, posttreatment: Showing disappearance of the lesion.

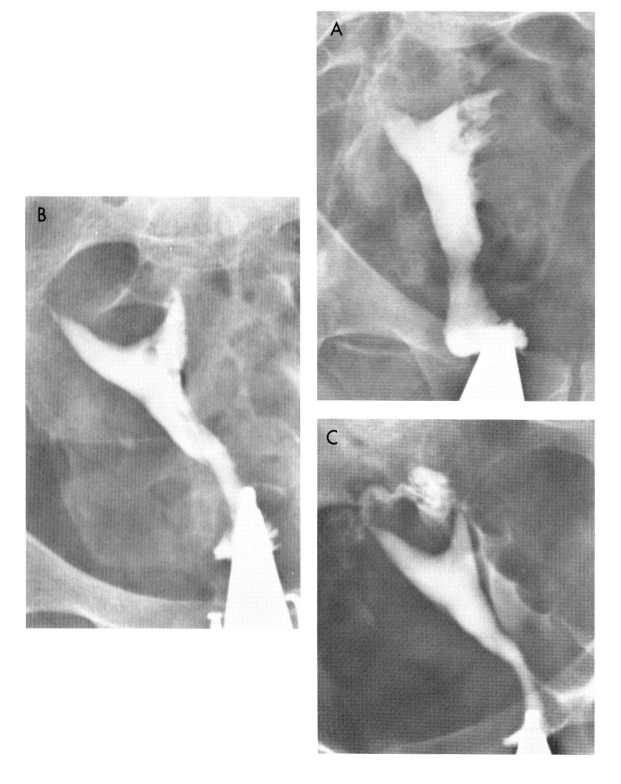

Figure 37 · Uterine Carcinoma: Treatment Response / 91

Figure 38.—Uterine carcinoma: failure of response due to extrauterine radium placement.

Control hysterogram, right posterior oblique projection, one month after first intracavitary radium treatment. The uterine cavity is expanded by a very large, undifferentiated cancer which looks surprisingly unaffected by therapy. At the level of the isthmus on the right (**arrow**) is a large cylindrical canal characteristic of mechanical perforation.

Comment: A control series of hysterograms will show not only regression of the tumor but lack of response to treatment. In this case the uterus was perforated and the radium inserted in an extrauterine position. The radiologist must be conversant with this picture because it can often explain an unexpected lack of response to treatment.

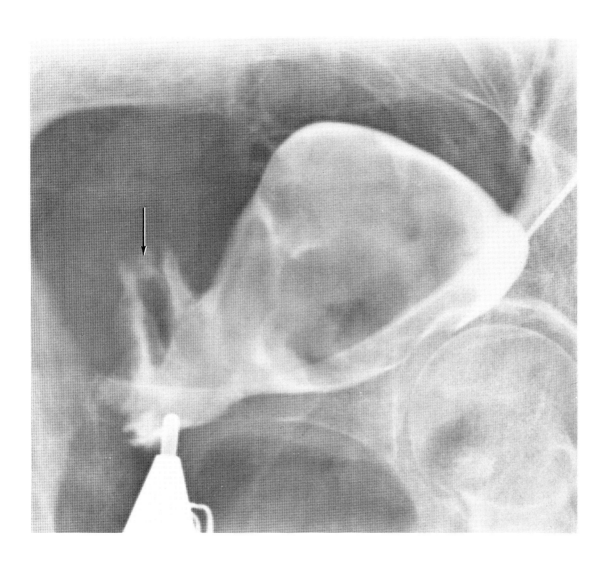

Figure 38 · Uterine Carcinoma: Treatment Response / 93

Figure 39.—Mixed mesodermal tumor of the uterus.

Anteroposterior projection: Showing a massive pelvic tumor extending into the upper abdomen. The ureters are displaced but not obstructed. Scattered calcifications (not unlike the picture in uterine fibroids) are seen in the upper abdomen (**arrows**). Such calcification is not uncommon in cartilaginous elements in this tumor.

The patient, age 53, was known to have an abdominal mass for many years but had refused surgery. Heavy vaginal bleeding had occurred and the mass now extended from the pelvis to the upper abdomen. An 8 × 12 in. uterine mass identified as a mixed mesodermal tumor was discovered at surgery. Many peritoneal and omental implants were noted. The patient died three months later.

Figure 39, courtesy of Dr. G. D. Dodd, M. D. Anderson Hospital, Houston, Tex.

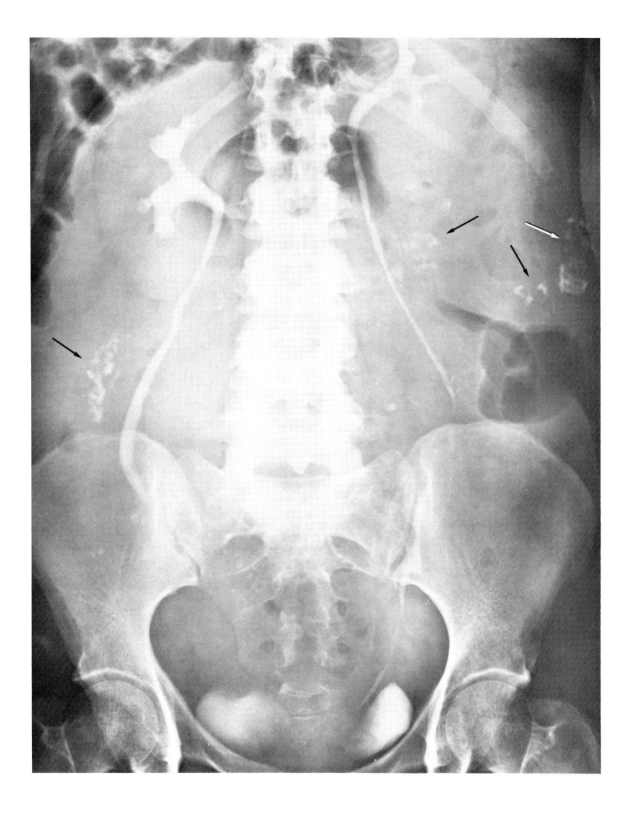

Figure 39 · Mixed Mesodermal Uterine Tumor / 95

Pelvic Angiography in Diagnosis of Extension and Recurrence of Carcinoma of the Cervix

SINCE CARCINOMA OF THE CERVIX is accessible for biopsy or cytologic examination, radiologic diagnosis has no role in the identification of the primary tumor. The inherent inaccuracies in clinical staging and in identifying recurrences after radiation therapy or surgery present a different problem, however, and in these situations pelvic angiography has played an increasingly important role. Among the most experienced advocates of this technique are Breit,[1] Lang and Greer[2] and Meng and Elkin.[3]

Since one is interested only in the hypogastric circulation most workers have chosen to inject contrast medium above the aortic bifurcation using an end-occluding catheter or to employ bilateral hypogastric selective catheterization. Difference of opinion exists as to the necessity of femoral artery occlusion in the inguinal region. The general technique of pelvic angiography is described on page 8; normal pelvic angiograms are shown in Figure 5.

The arteriographic features of cervical carcinoma are abnormal corkscrew vessels, tumor stain in the late capillary phase, arterial encasement producing attenuation, displacement, splaying and/or shortening as well as early venous filling. Breit,[1] drawing on an experience with over 400 pelvic angiographic examinations in carcinoma of the cervix, stated that of primary tumors approximately 70% are hypervascular while of recurrent tumors of the cervix only 30% are hypervascular. Only when the arterial supply is increased, or rarely if hypovascular and arcuate deflection is present, is diagnosis possible (Fig. 44). Arclike displacement is not seen in postradiation fibrosis according to Breit and serves as a distinguishing feature. Other tumors, both benign and malignant, could, however, produce such an appearance.

The vascularity of carcinoma of the cervix may prove to be of prognostic

---

[1] Breit, A.: *Angiographie der Uterustumoren und ihrer Rezidive* (Stuttgart: Georg Thieme Verlag, 1967).

[2] Lang, E. K., and Greer, J. L.: The value of pelvic arteriography for the staging of carcinoma of the cervix, Radiology 92:1027, 1969.

[3] Meng, C-H., and Elkin, M.: Gynecologic angiography, Seminars Radiol. 4:267, 1969.

value and an aid in selecting those patients who are more likely to be resistant to radiation. Breit found that of 140 patients assessed the two year survival was more than twice as large among patients whose tumors had a hypervascular pattern as among those with a hypovascular appearance. Illustrations of the characteristic angiographic features follow.

Figure 40.—Carcinoma of the cervix, stage III, with left parametrial extension to pelvic wall: pelvic arteriograms.

A, arterial phase, 3 seconds after completion of the injection, antero-posterior projection: Delineating the uterine vessels. The left uterine artery (**4**) is shortened due to parametrial infiltration. A tumor stain (**a**) is seen in the cervix and left parametrium.

(*Continued* on page 100.)

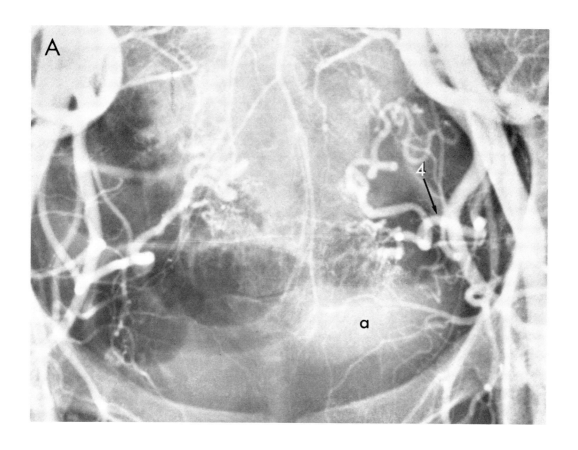

Figure 40 · Cervical Carcinoma with Extension / 99

Figure 40 (cont.).—Carcinoma of the cervix, stage III, with left parametrial extension to pelvic wall: pelvic arteriograms, left common iliac injection.

B, 1 second after completion of injection, anteroposterior view.

C, 2 seconds after completion of injection. A highly vascular tumor stain (**a**) is seen in the left parametrium.

D, 4 seconds after completion of injection. The large tumor stain (**a**) denotes the parametrial extension to the pelvic wall. Pelvic musculature (**arrow**) interposed between the tumor extension and the bony pelvis gives a "tumor-free" space.

E, drawing delineating uterine artery (**4**) and cervical vaginal branch (**5**) to the cervical carcinoma and left parametrial extension, as seen in **B, C** and **D.**

The patient, age 45, had a large exophytic squamous cell carcinoma of the cervix, stage III. The tumor arose in the left side of the cervix and extended into the left parametrium to the pelvic wall. (For further studies of this patient, see Figure 43.)

Figure 40, courtesy of Dr. A. Breit, Passau, W. Germany.

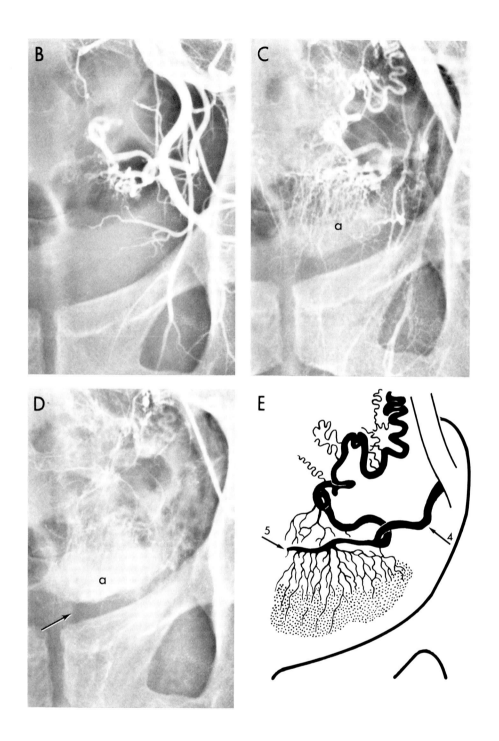

Figure 40 · Cervical Carcinoma with Extension / 101

Figure 41.—Recurrent carcinoma of the cervix with clinically undetectable metastasis to iliac region: pelvic arteriograms.

A, arterial phase, 2 seconds after completion of injection, anteroposterior projection: Showing compression of the right internal iliac artery (**a**), early tumor stain (**b**) and deformity of the inferior gluteal artery (**c**) on the right.

B, 3 seconds after completion of injection: Demonstrating a prominent tumor stain (**b**) on the right, in the area of the internal iliac artery with compression of its branches, and anastomosis of the sacral artery with the branches of the internal iliac artery (**d**).

C, drawing of **B,** delineating internal iliac artery (**2**), inferior gluteal artery (**3**), internal pudendal artery (**7**) and middle sacral artery (**9**).

The patient, age 60, had had radiation therapy for a stage II carcinoma of the cervix four years previously and was now suspected from her symptoms to have a recurrence, though no parametrial infiltration was clinically detectable.

(*Continued* on page 104.)

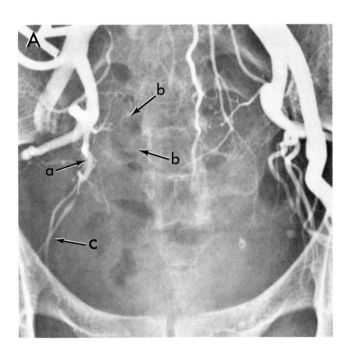

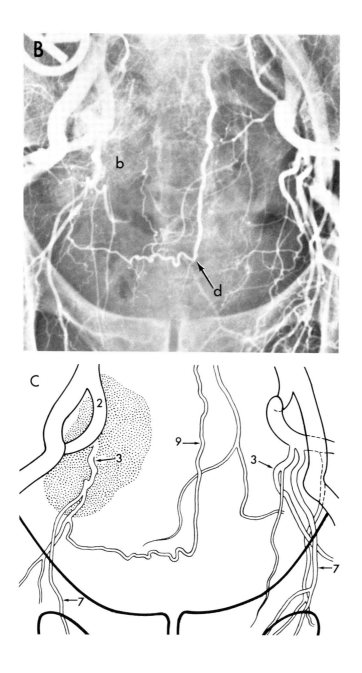

Figure 41 · Cervical Carcinoma with Metastasis / 103

Figure 41 (cont.).—Post-therapy arteriogram: recurrent carcinoma of the cervix with clinically undetectable metastasis to iliac region.

D, pelvic arteriogram following 5000 rads of cobalt-60; same arterial phase as in **B.** The tumor stain and right internal iliac artery compression have disappeared. The uterine arteries have now appeared on both sides; that on the right remains somewhat enlarged.

E, drawing of **D,** delineating external iliac artery (**1**), internal iliac artery (**2**), inferior gluteal artery (**3**), uterine artery (**4**), vaginal artery (**6**) and internal pudendal artery (**7**).

Comment: About 30% of the recurrences of carcinoma of the cervix are of the vascular type. In these cases the diagnosis is not generally difficult. In those of avascular type, recognition of recurrent tumor is often difficult if not impossible.

Figure 41, courtesy of Dr. A. Breit, Passau, W. Germany.

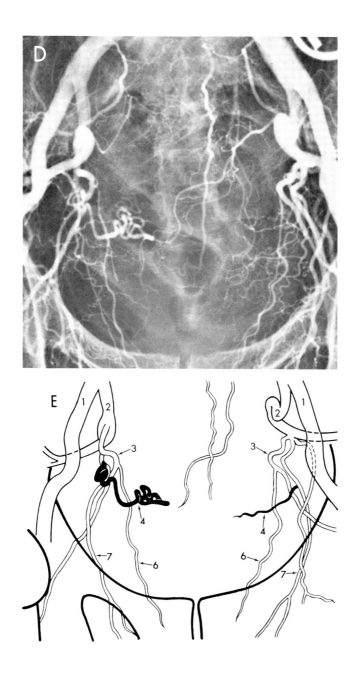

Figure 41 · Cervical Carcinoma with Metastasis / 105

Figure 42.—Highly vascularized stage III cervical carcinoma with extension to pelvic wall and upper vagina: pelvic arteriograms.

A, 1½ seconds after completion of injection; anteroposterior projection. The uterine artery is narrowed (**a**). There is early visualization of the uterine vessels, with tumor stain in the cervix and parametrial area (**b**). The uterus is retroflexed.

B, 2½ seconds after completion of injection. Tumor vessels extend to the pubic bone and into the upper vagina (**c**).

C, drawing of **B,** showing external iliac artery (**1**), internal iliac artery (**2**), inferior gluteal artery (**3**), uterine artery (**4**), cervical vaginal branch (**5**), internal pudendal artery (**6**) and tumor area (**b**).

The patient, age 53, had an ulcerating, moderately differentiated squamous cell carcinoma of the cervix, stage III, with right parametrial extension to the pelvic wall and upper vagina.

Figure 42, courtesy of Dr. A. Breit, Passau, W. Germany.

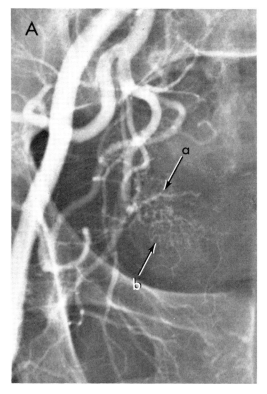

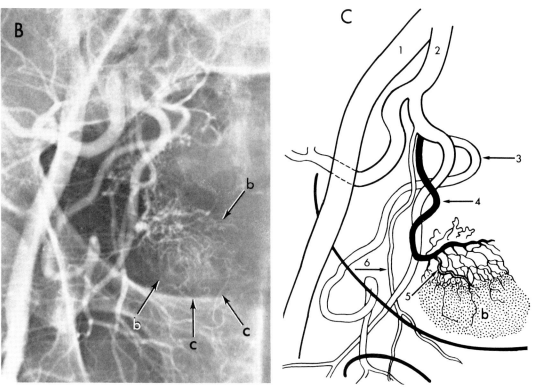

Figure 42 · Cervical Carcinoma with Extension / 107

Figure 43.—Cervical carcinoma before and after radiation therapy (same patient as in Fig. 40): pelvic arteriograms.

A, preoperative study 2 seconds after completion of injection, anteroposterior view: Showing tumor stain (**arrow**) in cervical and left parametrial area.

B, arteriogram following 6000 mg-hr. of radium therapy and 5000 rads of cobalt-60: Confirming marked reduction of tumor size and nearly complete disappearance of tumor vasculature.

The patient had stage III carcinoma of the cervix with left parametrial extension to the pelvic wall.

Comment: In general, very favorable tumor response has been noted in tumors as highly vascularized as this one.

Figure 43, courtesy of Dr. A. Breit, Passau, W. Germany.

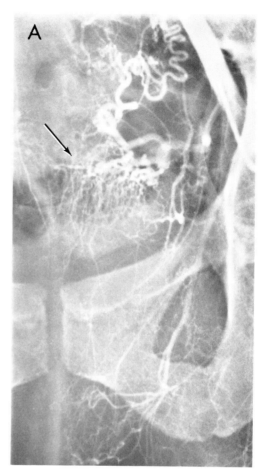

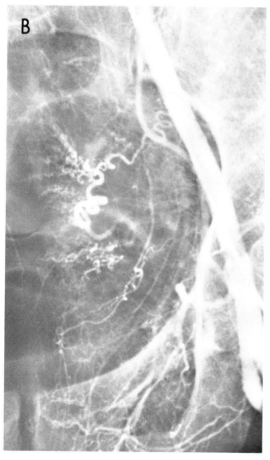

Figure 43 · Cervical Carcinoma: Treatment Response / 109

Figure 44.—Carcinoma of the cervix, stage III, hypovascular type: pelvic arteriograms.

A, arterial phase 1½ seconds after completion of injection, anteroposterior view. The uterine artery (**4** in **B**) is shortened and narrowed and the vaginal artery (**6**) is deflected in a smooth arc. Some extrinsic displacement of the left side of the bladder is evident.

B, drawing of **A,** delineating external iliac artery (**1**), internal iliac artery (**2**), inferior gluteal artery (**3**), uterine artery (**4**), vaginal branch (**6**), internal pudendal artery (**7**) and obturator artery (**8**).

C, late arterial phase 3 seconds after completion of injection: Showing no evidence of tumor stain or tumor vessels, only displacement.

The 46-year-old patient had a large stage III exophytic squamous cell carcinoma of the cervix which infiltrated the left parametrium.

Comment: About 30% of primary carcinomas of the cervix are poorly vascularized. The evidences of tumor (not specifically carcinoma of the cervix) include arterial deflection and vascular occlusion. Neither tumor stain nor tumor vessels are seen. The experience of some observers is that these are significantly less radiosensitive than highly vascular tumors.

Figure 44, courtesy of Dr. A. Breit, Passau, W. Germany.

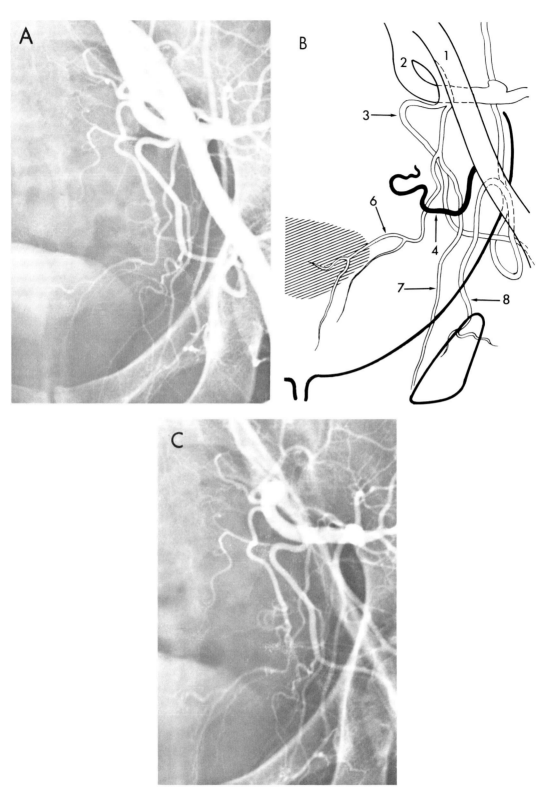

Figure 44 · Hypovascular Cervical Carcinoma / 111

Figure 45.—Carcinoma of the cervix with parametrial extension: pelvic arteriograms.

A, 1½ seconds after completion of injection, anteroposterior view. Normal blush of the uterine fundus is seen centrally (**a**), with some tumor vessels denoting tumor extension into the left parametrium (**b**).

B, 4½ second phase: Demonstrating blush of the left parametrial tumor extension (**b**). Note absence of a similar blush on the right.

This was a clinical stage Ic, grade III squamous cell carcinoma of the cervix corrected in staging by arteriography.

Figure 45, courtesy of Dr. E. K. Lang, Louisiana State University, Shreveport.

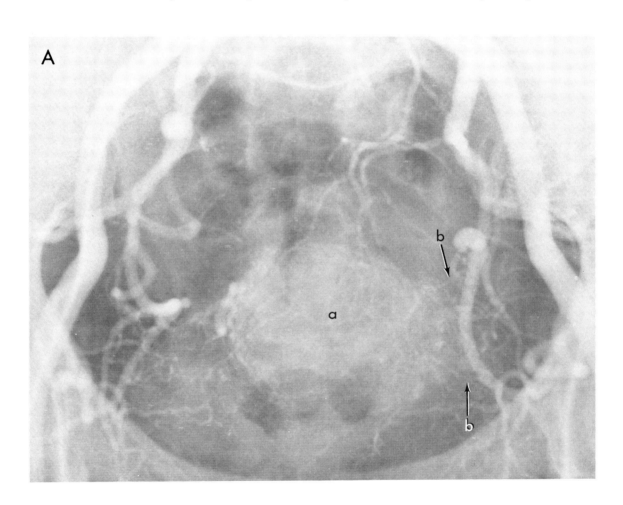

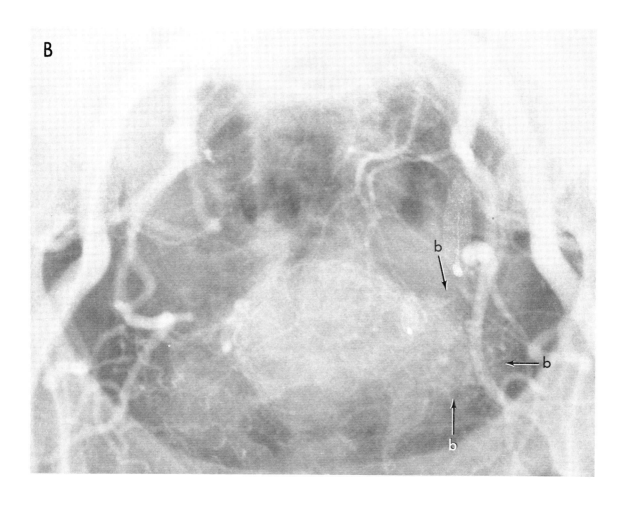

Figure 45 · Cervical Carcinoma with Extension / 113

Figure 46.—Stage IV cervical carcinoma: pelvic arteriograms.

A, selective left hypogastric arteriogram, early arterial (1 second) phase, anteroposterior view: Showing atheromatous plaques in hypogastric artery (**arrows**) and air-filled urinary bladder (**b**).

B, 7 second phase: Demonstrating extensive neovascularity and a dense stain extending into the left parametrium (**x**).

C, 11 second phase: Showing tumor extension to the left lateral parametrial wall.

This was a clinical stage IV, grade III squamous cell carcinoma. Selective catheterization of the left hypogastric artery was via the right femoral approach.

Figure 46, courtesy of Dr. E. K. Lang, Louisiana State University, Shreveport.

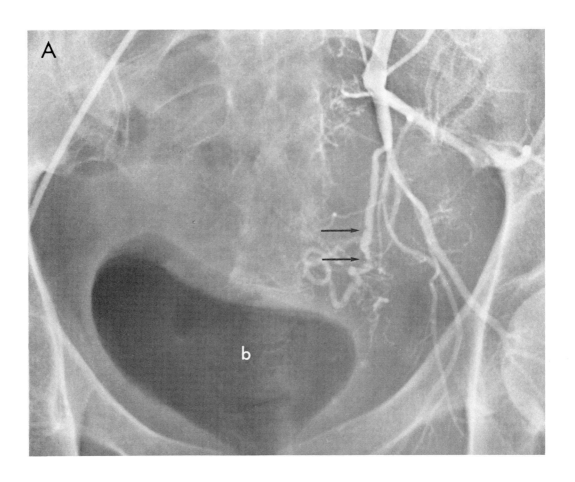

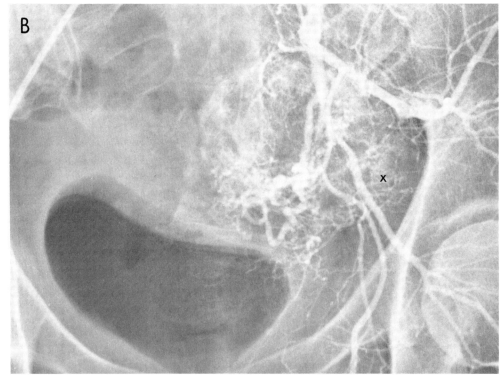

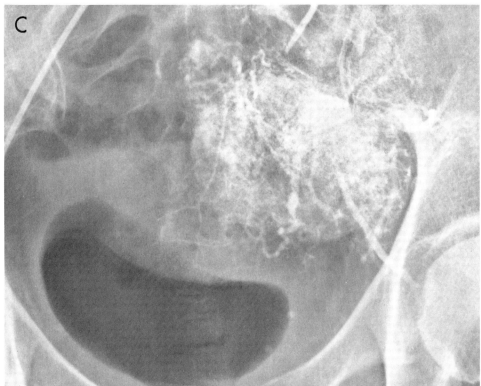

Figure 46 · Cervical Carcinoma / 115

Figure 47.—Carcinoma of the cervix: pelvic arteriograms.

A, 1½ second interval, anteroposterior view. Note extrinsic pressure effect on the right side of the dome of the gas-filled bladder (**arrows**).

B, 8 second interval: Revealing a large irregular dense tumor stain (**arrows**) in the right lower pelvis. The tumor extends to the right pelvic wall into the fornix and the vesical-vaginal septum (confirmed on surgical exploration).

This was a clinical stage IIb, grade II squamous cell carcinoma of the cervix. Pelvic arteriography was performed for assistance in staging.

Figure 47, courtesy of Dr. E. K. Lang, Louisiana State University, Shreveport.

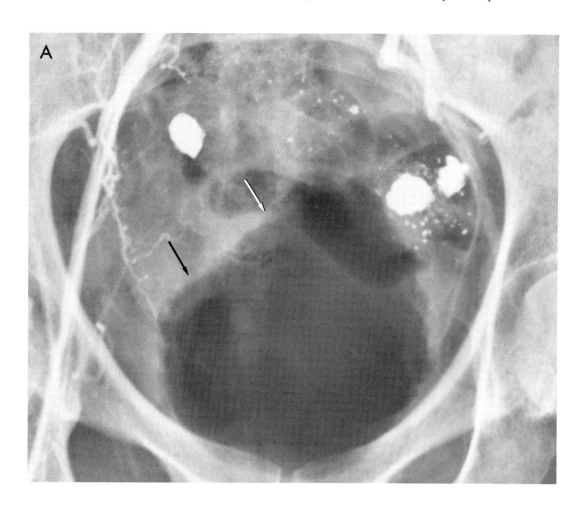

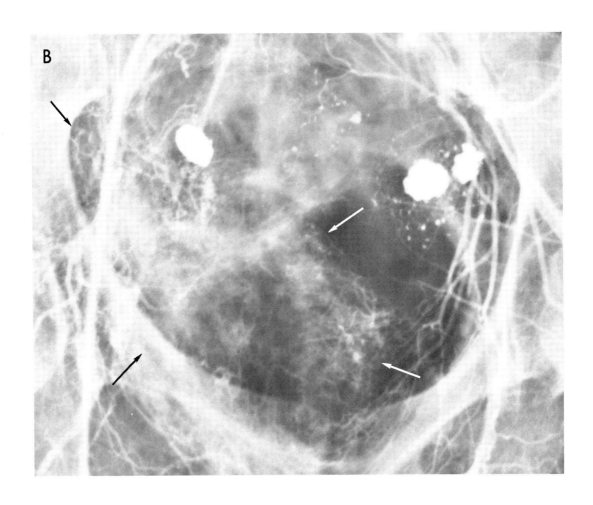

Figure 47 · Cervical Carcinoma with Extension / 117

Trophoblastic Tumors

HYDATIDIFORM MOLE, invasive mole and choriocarcinoma all are considered tumors of the placental trophoblast and occur following conception. Though they are uncommon or rare tumors they have radiologic importance which outweighs their frequency.

HYDATIDIFORM MOLE

This generally occurs as a proliferative process of trophoblastic tissue and hydropic degeneration of villous stroma following abortion in the earliest weeks of pregnancy. On occasion a mole may develop in association with a viable fetus. The frequency of hydatidiform mole in the United States is 1 per 2000–2500 pregnancies; its incidence is 10–30 times higher elsewhere in the world. The clinical indications of molar pregnancy include vaginal bleeding, absence of palpable fetal parts, inaudible heart sounds, larger uterus than is consistent with the duration of pregnancy, elevation of chorionic gonadotropin levels and the absence of fetal structure on radiography.

Once a mole is suspected and plain films show an unexpectedly large uterus and no fetal skeleton, two radiologic methods of investigation are useful, amniography and pelvic arteriography.

AMNIOGRAPHY.—The technique of amniography and its utility in diagnosing hydatidiform mole was described first by Bayan and Apelo[1] in 1957. Since then only minor modifications have been introduced. As pointed out by Wilson *et al.*,[2] this procedure has been incorrectly termed amniography in molar detection since the amnionic sac is generally small and the contrast agent is usually injected in the intervillous space. Common usage prevents discard of the term, however. After voiding to decompress the bladder, local anesthesia is established to the level of the peritoneum, several centimeters below the level of the umbilicus in the midline. A spinal type needle is satisfactory. Wilson *et al.*[2] have suggested the use of a needle polyethylene catheter assembly with a curl set in the tip of the catheter to prevent its inadvertent dislodgement during abdominal contraction after the needle has entered the intervillous space. After the needle is withdrawn from the catheter

---

[1] Bayan, F., and Apelo, R.: The direct and positive diagnosis of hydatidiform mole: A preliminary report, Philippine J. Surg. 12:1, 1957.

[2] Wilson, G.; Colodny, S., and Weidner, W.: Comparison of amniography and pelvic angiography in the diagnosis of hydatidiform mole, Radiology 87:1076, 1966.

the latter may be safely left in place for contrast reinjection if necessary. One should not expect to aspirate blood or amnionic fluid.

Approximately 20 cc of Renografin or similar contrast medium is injected in the uterine cavity and immediate filming in the anteroposterior, oblique and lateral projections is accomplished (Figs. 48–52). The contrast medium is absorbed quite rapidly in the usual case.[3, 4]

ARTERIOGRAPHY.—Since pelvic arteriography was first adapted for the diagnosis of trophoblastic tumors by Borell, Fernström and Westman in 1955 the procedure has been used widely. Their experience was reported in a splendid monograph in 1966.[5] Additional authoritative reports of large experience with the method have been made by Cockshott[6] and Brewis and Bagshawe.[7] When the level of chorionic gonadotropin has been demonstrated to be abnormally high, angiography can be used in conjunction with histologic examination to distinguish the type of trophoblastic neoplasm (particularly in problem cases), to evaluate the possibility of invasive trophoblastic neoplasm following a molar pregnancy, to evaluate the results of therapy and to assess recurrences. Cockshott,[6] however, believes that angiography alone serves this purpose and that curettage is to be avoided except when radiologic uncertainty exists.

Technique.—Pelvic arteriography is performed as described on page 8 with the following variations. The catheter tip should be so placed at a level in the aorta that the ovarian arteries as well as the iliac arteries are filled. The filming interval recommended by those most experienced with the trophoblastic tumors varies from 5–14 films taken in 8–12 seconds. The sequence recommended by Brewis and Bagshawe[7] is 2/second for 4 seconds, 1/second for 4 seconds, 1/2 seconds for 2 seconds. It is necessary to obtain films 5–10 seconds after completion of the injection in order to obtain opacification of the intervillous spaces into which the hydropic villi (vesicles) protrude.

Arteriographic Features of Hydatidiform Mole.—Uterine and ovarian artery caliber is often enlarged and the spiral myometrial vessels are dilated. Increased separation of the uterine arteries is produced by uterine enlargement in some (Figs. 53 and 54). The normal irregular frayed contour of the

---

[3] Bayan, F., and Apelo, R.: The direct and positive diagnosis of hydatidiform mole: A preliminary report, Philippine J. Surg. 12:1, 1957.

[4] Wilson, G.; Colodny, S., and Weidner, W.: Comparison of amniography and pelvic angiography in the diagnosis of hydatidiform mole, Radiology 87:1076, 1966.

[5] Borell, U., *et al.: The Diagnosis of Hydatidiform Mole, Malignant Hydatidiform Mole and Choriocarcinoma with Special Reference to the Diagnostic Value of Pelvic Arteriography* (Springfield, Ill.: Charles C Thomas, Publisher, 1966).

[6] Cockshott, W. P.: Angiography in trophoblastic tumors, Seminars Radiol. 4:280, 1969.

[7] Brewis, R. A. L., and Bagshawe, K. D.: Pelvic arteriography in invasive trophoblastic neoplasia, Brit. J. Radiol. 41:481, 1968.

intervillous spaces in a normal pregnancy is altered by intrusion of hydropic villi (vesicles) which create crescentic, round or scalloped outlines in the intervillous spaces and diminish the number of these spaces which can be identified (Fig. 55). Because of the bulk of some lesions the contrast medium may become quite dilute, thus masking the diagnostic features unless more than 60 cc of contrast agent is used. At times, localized evidence of molar pregnancy is explained by the fact that only a few villi may be abnormal in a segment of otherwise normal placenta. There is no area of greatly increased vascular opacification over normal pregnancy, nor is there early venous filling in benign hydatidiform mole. Characteristic arteriographic features of molar pregnancy were identified in 11 of 12 patients studied by Borell *et al.*[8]

INVASIVE TROPHOBLASTIC NEOPLASMS

Invasive trophoblastic neoplasms (ITN), which include chorioadenoma destruens (invasive mole) and choriocarcinoma, are an uncommon complication following hydatidiform mole (one-third), abortion and ectopic pregnancy (one-third) and normal pregnancy (one-third). The frequency of choriocarcinoma is about 1 per 20,000–40,000 pregnancies in the United States. Because invasive hydatidiform mole and choriocarcinoma cannot generally be distinguished by pathologic criteria, hormonal assay or angiography alone they must, for practical purposes, be considered as one entity representing a spectrum of malignancy. Experience has proved that it is necessary to utilize the contributions of curettage, hormone assay and arteriography together to diagnose accurately the presence of this process in some instances. Since the introduction of antifolic acid therapy, invasive trophoblastic neoplasms have been treated with dramatically improved success and their recognition has become essential. The three recognized diagnostic methods each have advantages and shortcomings which are summarized here.

HUMAN CHORIONIC GONADOTROPIN (HCG) ASSAY.—Qualitative analysis of HCG, while easily available, lacks specificity and reliability. Although it may be a useful screening test in some circumstances if used repeatedly, it is unacceptable when compared with quantitative analysis.[9]

Quantitative HCG assay is far more complicated to perform and less commonly available but has become essential for the early diagnosis and proper management of trophoblastic neoplasms. The levels of HCG are

---

[8] Borell, U., *et al.: The Diagnosis of Hydatidiform Mole, Malignant Hydatidiform Mole and Choriocarcinoma with Special Reference to the Diagnostic Value of Pelvic Arteriography* (Springfield, Ill.: Charles C Thomas, Publisher, 1966).

[9] Venning, E. H.: Hormonal Physiology of the Placenta—Tropic Hormones and Steroid Metabolism, in Gold, J. J. (ed.): *Textbook of Gynecologic Endocrinology* (New York: Hoeber Med. Div., Harper & Row, 1968).

universally elevated in the presence of hydatidiform mole and invasive trophoblastic neoplasms. Because of this, hormonal assay is more important than histologic examination following curettement in detecting trophoblastic neoplasms.[10] Unfortunately the distinction between noninvasive and invasive trophoblastic disease cannot be made by this method alone.

Since the HCG level rapidly falls to normal within 48 hours following normal delivery or termination of pregnancy, a sustained level or rise must be viewed with concern. Brewer et al.[11] found that within 60 days following termination of a molar pregnancy serial chorionic gonadotropin titers had returned to normal in 70% of patients. Most of the remainder are assumed to have invasive mole or choriocarcinoma and are given prophylactic chemotherapy.

As time has passed and the methods of quantitative HCG assay have improved, greater reliance has been placed on hormone assay for the detection of invasive trophoblastic neoplasm and less dependence on arteriography has resulted.

CURETTAGE.—Because curettings often do not include myometrial tissue it is frequently impossible to determine the invasiveness of a tumor and to classify it precisely. When ITN is extrauterine or intramural, endometrial curettings are sure to be nondiagnostic or misleading. On the other hand, when curettement reveals large amounts of trophoblastic tissue and definite evidence of neoplasia with no evidence of villi, there is little doubt of malignancy. Curettage incurs the additional hazards of tumor embolization through the rich vasculature of the tumor and the possibility of massive hemorrhage.

PELVIC ARTERIOGRAPHY.—Enthusiasm for the use of pelvic arteriography varies from those who routinely use this procedure to those who never do, the latter relying exclusively on quantitative HCG assay. Arteriography is unnecessary in every case but would seem to be particularly helpful in (1) distinguishing between retained mole and invasive trophoblastic neoplasm in problem cases, (2) assisting in the earlier detection of invasive tumors in patients whose HCG levels remain elevated after molar pregnancy and (3) determining the feasibility of hypogastric infusion therapy which allows a much lower and less toxic chemotherapy dose in patients with refractory or localized tumors.[12]

---

[10] Novak, E. R., and Woodruff, J. D.: *Novak's Gynecologic and Obstetric Pathology, With Clinical and Endocrine Relations* (6th ed.; Philadelphia: W. B. Saunders Company, 1967).

[11] Brewer, J. I., *et al.*: Hydatidiform mole: A follow-up regimen for identification of invasive mole and choriocarcinoma and for selection of patients for treatment, Am. J. Obst. & Gynec. 101:557, 1968.

[12] Epstein, D. N.: The Management of Gestational Trophoblastic Disease, in Sturgis, S. S.,

Dependence on arteriography to judge the effectiveness of chemotherapy is handicapped by two facts. (1) Invasive trophoblastic neoplasm can regress in the pelvis while distant metastases persist. (2) Arteriovenous fistulas, which in some respects simulate the vascular spaces in invasive tumors, may remain after successful chemotherapy.[13] Brewis and Bagshawe,[16] in a large experience with angiography, found no example of diagnostic arteriographic features when the HCG was not elevated. Some ITN tumors, on the other hand, had so little vascularity that the arteriographic diagnosis could not be made.

Angiographic Features of Invasive Trophoblastic Neoplasm.—In the more malignant tumors, ovarian and uterine arteries are generally enlarged and the spiral intramural arteries feed directly into amorphous vascular spaces (Figs. 56–63). Such spaces are usually intrauterine but at times may be extrauterine. Contrast persists in these spaces for variable lengths of time, ranging from delayed egress to exceptionally rapid disappearance into venous channels, which in essence constitute arteriovenous fistulas (Fig. 58). Within the center of the vascular spaces approximately 40% of the patients with ITN will show central radiolucency due to old blood clot and amorphous fibrinoid material.[16] The periphery is composed of actively growing tumor. Extrauterine deposits of tumor may have the same features (Fig. 61). An additional, though less specific feature, of ITN is increased size and visibility of intramural arteries and veins, particularly in the vicinity of the tumor (Figs. 58 and 59).

The arteriographic pattern of trophoblastic tumors must be differentiated from normal pregnancy, early ectopic pregnancy, missed abortion and placenta accreta. This is not always easy or possible.[14–16] Generally, however, the combination of history, physical findings, serial HCG assay, curettage and angiography will differentiate these entities.[13]

SURVEY FOR METASTASIS.—Certain circumstances require a careful search for metastasis (Figs. 64 and 65). When further pregnancies are not desired, some favor hysterectomy for the treatment of ITN if disease is localized to the uterus. In others the consideration of surgical removal or localized chemoperfusion of disease which is refractory to therapy requires

and Traymor, M. H. (eds.): *Progress in Gynecology* (New York: Grune & Stratton, Inc., 1969), Vol. V, p. 397.

[13] Cockshott, W. P., and Hendrickse, J. P. deV.: Persistent arteriovenous fistulae following the chemotherapy of malignant trophoblastic disease, Radiology 88:329, 1967.

[14] Borell, U., *et al.: The Diagnosis of Hydatidiform Mole, Malignant Hydatidiform Mole and Choriocarcinoma with Special Reference to the Diagnostic Value of Pelvic Arteriography* (Springfield, Ill.: Charles C Thomas, Publisher, 1966).

[15] Cockshott, W. P.: Angiography in trophoblastic tumors, Seminars Radiol. 4:280, 1969.

[16] Brewis, R. A. L., and Bagshawe, K. D.: Pelvic arteriography in invasive trophoblastic neoplasia, Brit. J. Radiol. 41:481, 1968.

identification of metastasis. For this purpose chest radiography, hepatic arteriography, brain scan and EEG should be carried out.[17] It should be remembered that pulmonary metastases frequently regress initially following chemotherapy, then persist unchanged long after HCG titers have returned to normal because of tumor replacement by fibrous tissue.

---

[17] Epstein, D. N.: The Management of Gestational Trophoblastic Disease, in Sturgis, S. S., and Traymor, M. H. (eds.): *Progress in Gynecology* (New York: Grune & Stratton, Inc., 1969), Vol. V, p. 397.

Figure 48.—Hydatidiform mole: amniogram.

Anteroposterior projection: Demonstrating rounded hydropic villi (vesicles) typical of hydatidiform mole.

An unmarried 18-year-old patient who was three months pregnant sought a therapeutic abortion. This procedure was recommended by the Therapeutic Abortion Committee and hypertonic saline amniocentesis was planned. Rather than obtaining amnionic fluid, only blood was aspirated. A mole was suspected and amniography performed. Vacuum curettage followed, then sharp curettement with removal of a typical hydatidiform mole.

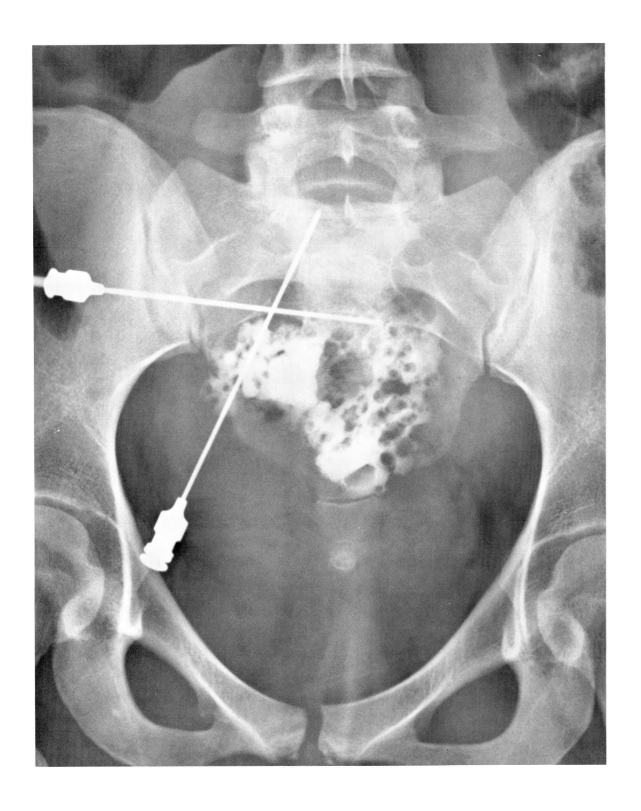

Figure 48 · Hydatidiform Mole: Amniography / 125

Figure 49.—Hydatidiform mole: amniograms.

A, anteroposterior view: Showing multiple small rounded radiolucencies corresponding to hydatidiform vesicles surrounded by contrast medium (**x**).

B, oblique projection: Revealing characteristic hydatidiform vesicles (**x**).

The 17-year-old gravida I, para 0 patient complained of vaginal spotting and shortness of breath. According to the history she was 16 weeks pregnant, though the uterus was enlarged to 22 week size. No fetal heart tones were audible, nor were fetal parts palpable or visible on a plain film. Chorionic gonadotropin level was elevated to 1.6 million units.

Figure 49, courtesy of Dr. G. Wilson, University of California at Los Angeles Medical Center, Los Angeles.

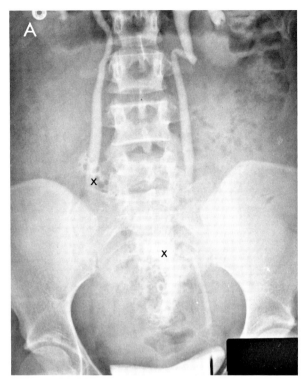

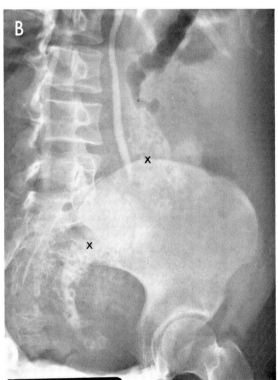

Figure 49 · Hydatidiform Mole: Amniography / 127

Figure 50.—Hydatidiform mole: amniogram.

Anteroposterior projection: Demonstrating innumerable small vesicles (**x**) typical of hydatidiform mole.

The 19-year-old gravida V, para 3 patient who was 14 weeks pregnant according to the history was admitted with a complaint of severe nausea and vomiting and vaginal bleeding. The uterine enlargement was consistent with a 20 week gestation. The HCG level was 6 million units. There were no signs of fetal viability. After evacuation of the mole, the HCG level gradually fell to normal in six weeks.

Figure 50, courtesy of Dr. G. Wilson, University of California at Los Angeles Medical Center, Los Angeles.

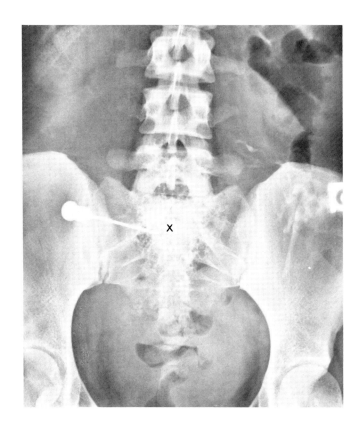

Figure 50 · Hydatidiform Mole: Amniography / 129

Figure 51.—Hydatidiform mole: amniograms.

A, anteroposterior projection: Showing most of the contrast medium in intervillous spaces and many vesicles of varying size (**a**). There is an oval collection of contrast apparently in the chorionic sac (**b**).

B, delayed film. Contrast has rapidly disappeared from the intervillous spaces and is being excreted by the kidneys. The contrast in the chorionic sac remains (**b**).

At age 18 this patient was seen in the emergency room with slight vaginal bleeding. By estimation from her last menstrual period she was 14 weeks pregnant, yet uterine enlargement was consistent with an 18 or 19 week pregnancy. A plain film of the abdomen demonstrated no fetal skeleton.

Figure 51, courtesy of Dr. J. J. McCort, Valley Medical Center, San Jose, Calif.

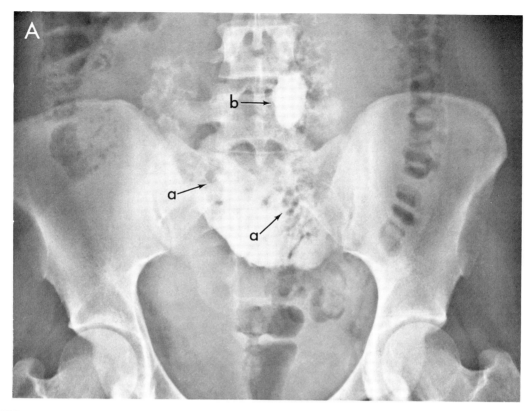

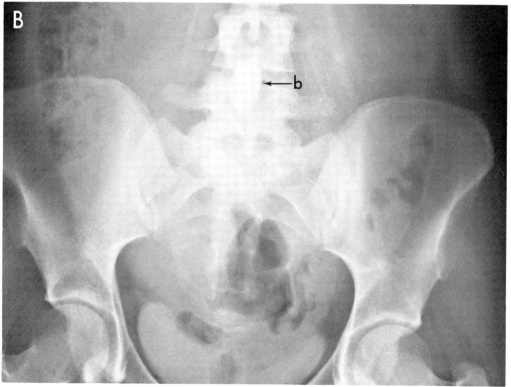

Figure 51 · Hydatidiform Mole: Amniography / 131

Figure 52.—Hydatidiform mole: amniograms.

A, anteroposterior projection. Contrast in the intervillous spaces delineates villous vesicles of varying size (**a**) in a hydatidiform mole. Most of the medium is apparently in the chorionic sac (**b**).

B, lateral view: Delineating villous vesicles (**a**) and chorionic sac (**b**).

A 17-year-old gravida III, para 2 patient in the fourteenth week of pregnancy entered the hospital with profuse vaginal bleeding. The uterus was the size of a 20 week pregnancy. The HCG titer was 1.6 million units.

Comment: The uterine cavity in this condition is filled with grapelike villous vesicles which distort the amnionic sac. Because the embryo is nonviable, the amnionic and chorionic sacs are much smaller than normal.

Figure 52, *A,* courtesy of Wilson, G., *et al.:* Radiology 87:1076, 1966; *B,* courtesy of Dr. G. Wilson, University of California at Los Angeles Medical Center, Los Angeles.

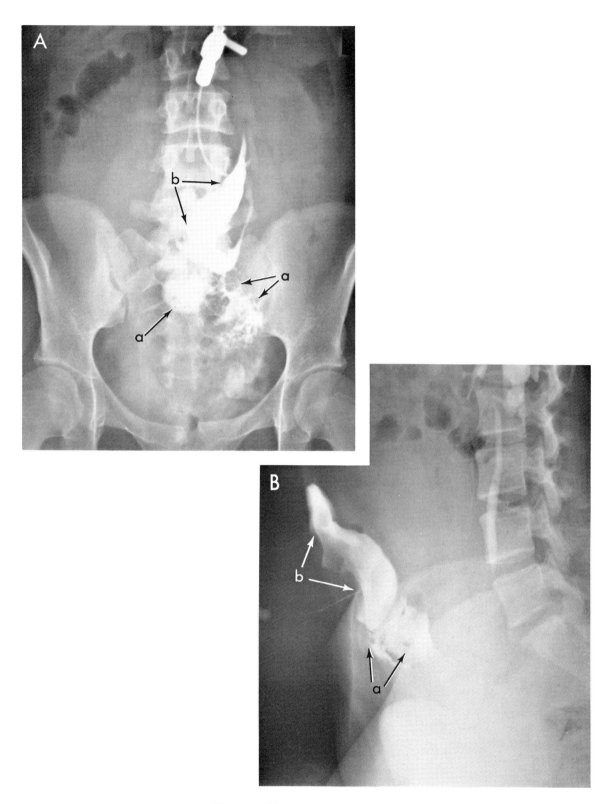

Figure 52 · Hydatidiform Mole: Amniography / 133

Figure 53.—Hydatidiform mole: pelvic angiograms.

A, arterial phase, anteroposterior view: Gross uterine enlargement indicated by separation of enlarged uterine arteries (**a**). The arterial phase is nonspecific.

B, late venous phase: Hydropic villous vesicles related to molar pregnancy (**x**) displace contrast medium in intervillous spaces.

A woman, 40, with uterine enlargement inconsistent with the stage of her pregnancy and absence of fetal heart sounds was studied angiographically for suspected molar pregnancy.

Comment: The late phase films taken 5–10 seconds after completion of the injection best show the evidence of hydatidiform mole.

Figure 53, *A,* courtesy of Dr. K. D. Bagshawe, Charing Cross and Fulham Hospitals, London; *B,* courtesy of Brewis, R. A. L., and Bagshawe, K. D.: Brit. J. Radiol. 41:481, 1968.

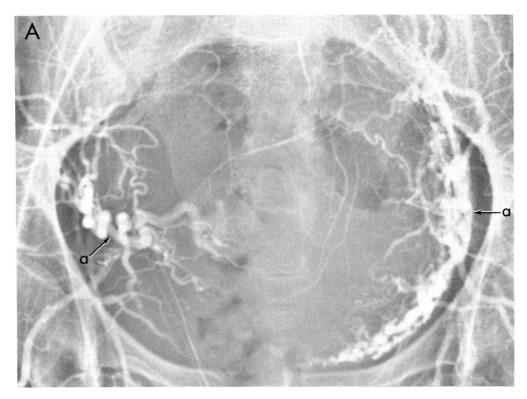

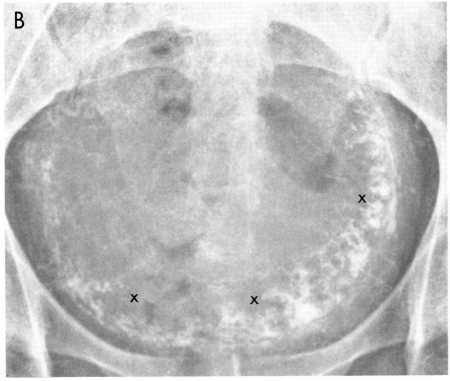

Figure 53 · Hydatidiform Mole: Pelvic Angiography / 135

Figure 54.—Hydatidiform mole: pelvic angiograms.

A, arterial phase, anteroposterior projection: Delineating enlarged and widely separated uterine arteries (**a**) due to uterine enlargement, and dilated spiral myometrial arteries (**b**).

B, late venous phase: Showing contrast medium in intervillous spaces displaced by hydropic vesicles of molar pregnancy, creating multiple circular and arcuate filling defects (**x**).

A 36-year-old woman in the twenty-third week of pregnancy had vaginal spotting and uterine enlargement greater than expected for the duration of gestation. No fetal skeleton was observed. Angiography was performed and curettage confirmed the presence of benign mole.

Figure 54, courtesy of Drs. C. Rådberg and I. Wickbom, Gothenberg, Sweden.

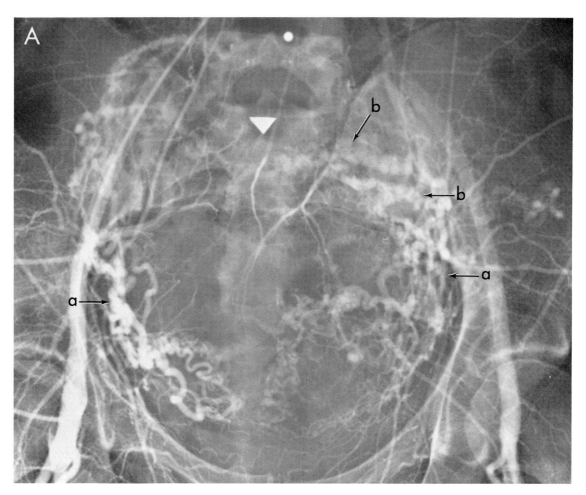

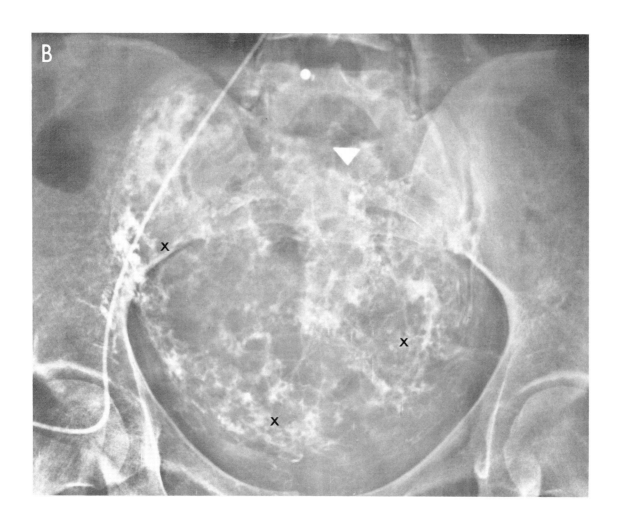

Figure 54 · Hydatidiform Mole: Pelvic Angiography / 137

Figure 55.—Hydatidiform mole: pelvic angiogram.

Late phase, anteroposterior exposure: Showing hydropic villi in the lower part of the uterine cavity (**x**).

A gravida IV, para 3 woman of 39 had uterine enlargement to the size of a term pregnancy, absence of fetal life signs, dyspnea, proteinuria and blood pressure 190/105. The HCG level was 5 million units.

Comment: Because of marked uterine enlargement and dilution of contrast medium in the intervillous spaces, the contrast may become quite dilute unless the standard bolus is increased to approximately 60 cc.

Figure 55, courtesy of Dr. K. D. Bagshawe, Charing Cross and Fulham Hospitals, London.

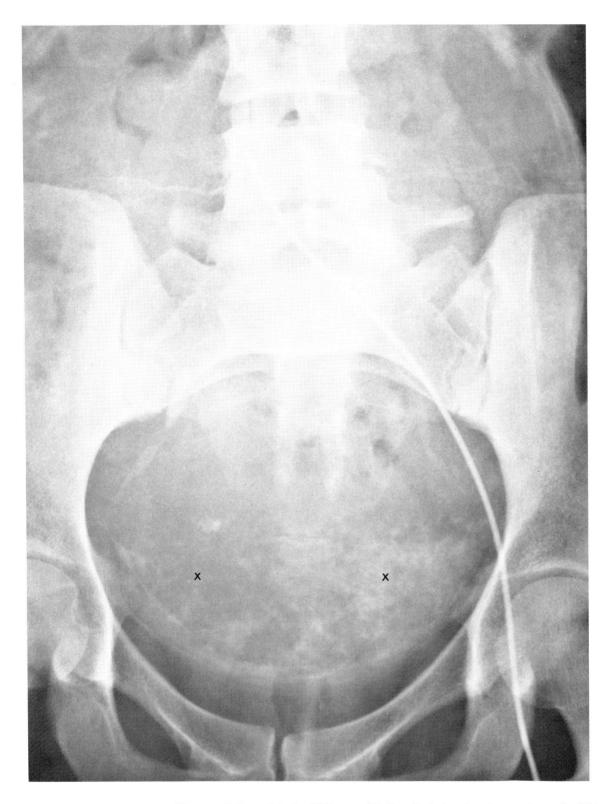

Figure 55 · Hydatidiform Mole: Pelvic Angiography / 139

Figure 56.—Postmolar invasive trophoblastic neoplasm, emphasizing occasional inconsistency of angiographic and clinical appearance: pelvic angiograms.

March, 1965:

A, late arterial phase, anteroposterior view: showing intramural arteries greatly increased in number and size, and small intramural cavity (**a**). The HCG level was just above normal at this time.

B, early venous phase. Contrast in the small cavity persists (**a**). Enlarged intramural veins (**b**).

A woman of 26 had a miscarriage at 5 months during her first pregnancy.
September, 1964.—Second pregnancy; hydatidiform mole.
November, 1964.—Molar vesicles passed.
December, 1964.—Urinary HCG excretion 5000 units per day. Pelvic angiography showed enlarged hypervascular uterus. Gonadotropin excretion rate was falling so no therapy was given.
March–September, 1965.—Repeat angiograms showed progressive dilatation of uterine vessels. Throughout this period, HCG excretion remained just above normal and the patient had oligomenorrhea.
March, 1966.—Pelvic angiography showed no abnormality but the HCG level was rising. Vaginal bleeding started. Curettage was negative. The patient was then treated with methotrexate and folinic acid for three months.
December, 1968.—She was well and HCG excretion normal.

Comment: This case illustrates the occasional inconsistency between angiographic appearance and biologic activity as reflected by HCG assay. At the time of normal angiography in March, 1966, the neoplasm was again active, though not necessarily in the pelvis.

Figure 56, courtesy of Dr. K. D. Bagshawe, Charing Cross and Fulham Hospitals, London.

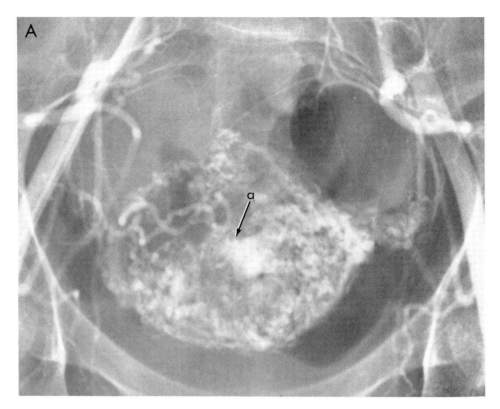

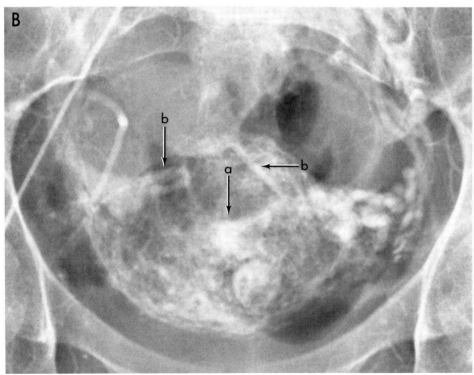

Figure 56 · Invasive Trophoblastic Neoplasm / 141

Figure 57.—Invasive hydatidiform mole: pelvic arteriogram.

Arteriogram following completion of chemotherapy, anteroposterior view. The uterus remains enlarged and villous vesicles are seen in the right side (**a**). Intramural tributaries of the uterine artery are very large; some enter ill-defined vascular spaces (**b**), but no early venous filling is seen.

May 16.—First pregnancy. Hydatidiform mole evacuated. Continued vaginal bleeding, enlarged uterus and positive pregnancy test.

June 27.—Curettings contained hyperplastic trophoblasts. The HCG excretion remained abnormal after nine courses of methotrexate and three of actinomycin D.

July 12.—Pelvic arteriography (shown here) was performed. Because of its appearance choriocarcinoma could not be excluded.

October 19.—Hysterectomy revealed a large part of the anterior uterine wall replaced by invasive mole.

Comment: Rounded radiolucent filling defects suggesting hydropic vesicles are present on occasion in choriocarcinoma so do not always exclude this possibility.

Figure 57, courtesy of Dr. K. D. Bagshawe, Charing Cross and Fulham Hospitals, London.

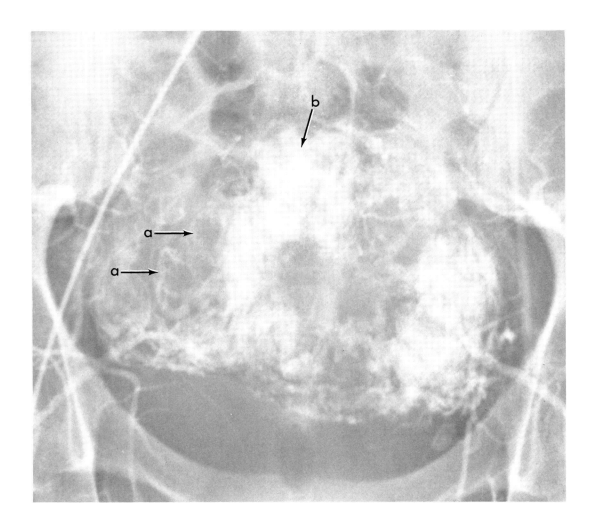

Figure 57 · Invasive Trophoblastic Neoplasm / 143

Figure 58.—Postmolar invasive trophoblastic neoplasm: pelvic arteriograms.

A, early phase, anteroposterior projection: The uterine artery feeds into intramural vascular spaces (**a**) and immediately into uterine veins (**b**), constituting an arteriovenous shunt in the right side of the uterus.

B, late arterial phase: Small spiral intramural arteries (**arrow**) remain filled in the left side of the uterus while massive shunting and extensive venous filling are evident on the right (**x**).

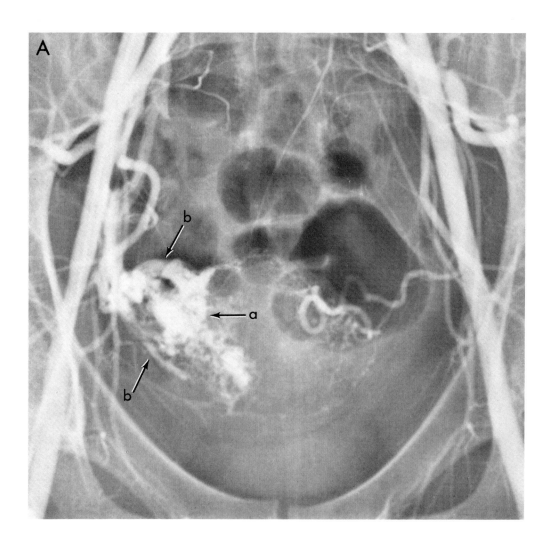

The patient, age 27, had a hydatidiform mole evacuated by Pitocin infusion followed by curettage. For the next seven weeks she had continuous bleeding and/or brown discharge. She was hospitalized with weight loss, anorexia and right iliac fossa pain and tenderness. Urinary HCG excretion was 8000 units a day. After pelvic arteriography, she was given intra-aortic methotrexate infusion and intermittent intramuscular folinic acid injections in four courses. She was well, with normal HCG excretion, five years later.

Figure 58, courtesy of Dr. K. D. Bagshawe, Charing Cross and Fulham Hospitals, London.

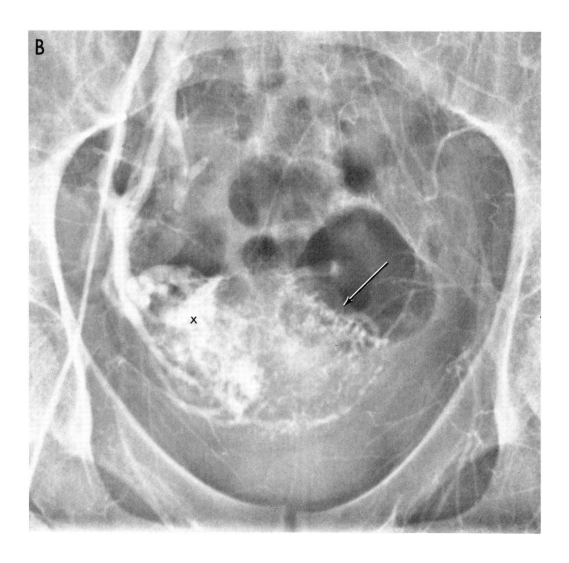

Figure 58 · Invasive Trophoblastic Neoplasm / 145

Figure 59.—Postmolar invasive trophoblastic neoplasm: pelvic arteriograms.

A, early arterial phase, anteroposterior view: Revealing enlarged uterine arteries (**a**).

B, late arterial phase: Demonstrating some prominent uterine veins in the upper lateral aspect of the uterus (**b**) with drainage into the ovarian vein (**c**). An occasional vesicular villus is seen (**d**).

The patient, 20, during her first pregnancy spontaneously evacuated a hydatidiform mole in May, 1964. Subsequently she was asymptomatic and pregnancy tests were negative. From November to February, 1965, she had amenorrhea, and in mid-March pregnancy was suspected. Chest films showed

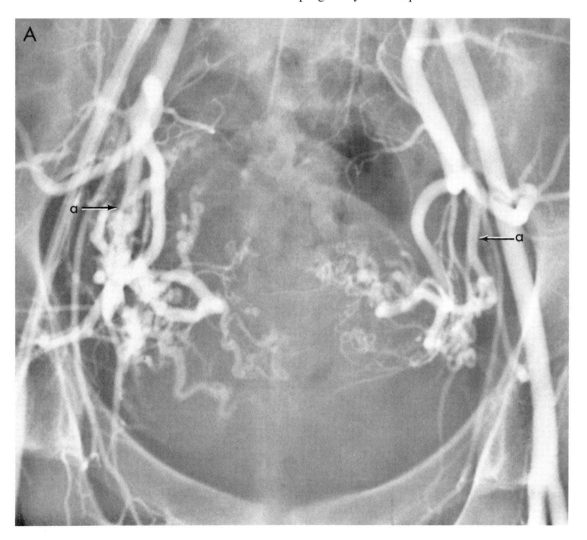

multiple opacities consistent with metastasis. Two days later there was vaginal bleeding, and in 10 days an irregular orange-size mass was palpable on the right side of the uterus on pelvic examination. Pelvic arteriography was performed at this time. Urinary HCG excretion was 2 million units a day. She was treated with methotrexate, 6-mercaptopurine and actinomycin D, and 19 months later was well with no evidence of residual disease. Subsequently she had a normal pregnancy.

Comment: Arteriography in this case was complementary to HCG assay in confirming diagnosis without resort to hysterectomy.

Figure 59, courtesy of Dr. K. D. Bagshawe, Charing Cross and Fulham Hospitals, London.

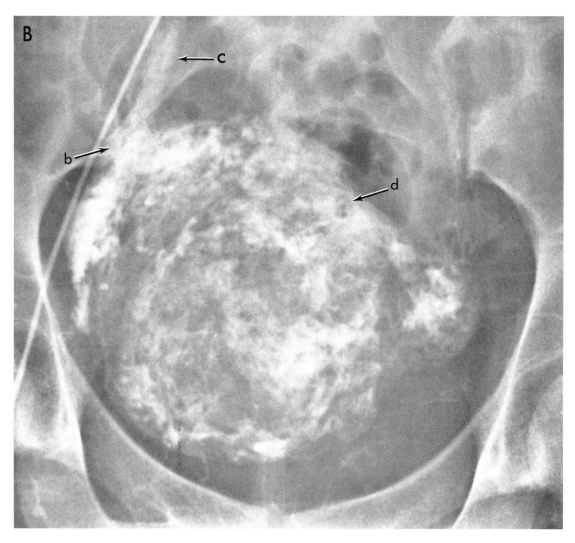

Figure 59 · Invasive Trophoblastic Neoplasm / 147

Figure 60.—Invasive trophoblastic neoplasm: angiograms.

A, early arterial phase, anteroposterior view: Showing enlarged uterine arteries (**a**) and enlarged, tortuous spiral intramural arteries (**b**).

B, later arterial phase: Showing vascular spaces (**c**) fed by spiral intramural arteries (**b**). Early filling of uterine veins (**d**) indicates arteriovenous shuntlike communication.

C, later arterial phase: Showing changing shape of vascular spaces (**c**) as series progresses, and persistent early venous filling (**d**).

A woman, 31, after expelling a hydatidiform mole continued to have HCG elevation. After angiography, curettage confirmed the presence of invasive trophoblastic neoplasm, probably choriocarcinoma. Methotrexate therapy was followed by hysterectomy, which showed no residual tumor.

Figure 60, courtesy of Drs. C. Rådberg and I. Wickbom, Gothenberg, Sweden.

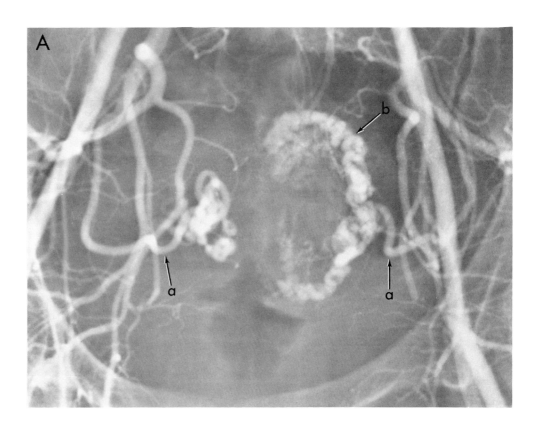

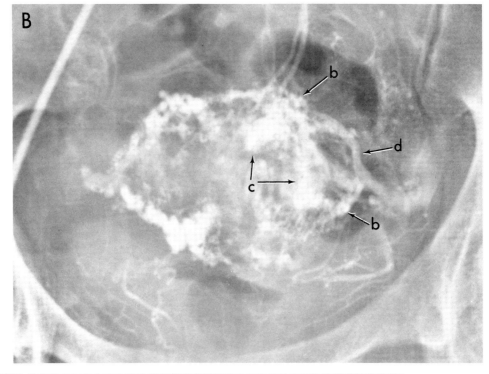

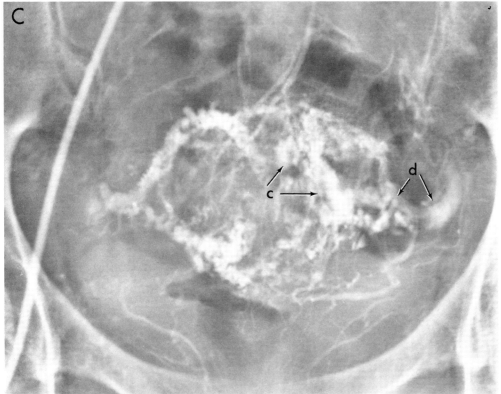

Figure 60 · Invasive Trophoblastic Neoplasm / 149

Figure 61.—Choriocarcinoma with parametrial and vaginal extension: pelvic angiogram.

Late arterial phase, anteroposterior view: Revealing large extrauterine vascular spaces in choriocarcinoma with extension into the left parametrium (**a**) and vagina (**b**).

A gravida II, para 1 woman, age 28, had spontaneous abortion in 1963, followed by hydatidiform mole in May, 1964. Thereafter the pregnancy test was alternately positive and negative until April, 1965, when heavy vaginal bleeding, urinary retention, dyspnea, hemoptysis and abdominal pain were present. On hospitalization, multiple pulmonary metastases were found; HCG excretion was 400,000 units a day. The angiogram shown here was obtained at this time. Four courses of chemotherapy followed, then pelvic laparotomy and hysterectomy because of persistent disease. The uterus was enlarged to the size of a 10 week pregnancy, and rectovaginal tumor extending into the vaginal vault was found. The tumor was not controlled and the patient died.

Figure 61, courtesy of Dr. K. D. Bagshawe, Charing Cross and Fulham Hospitals, London.

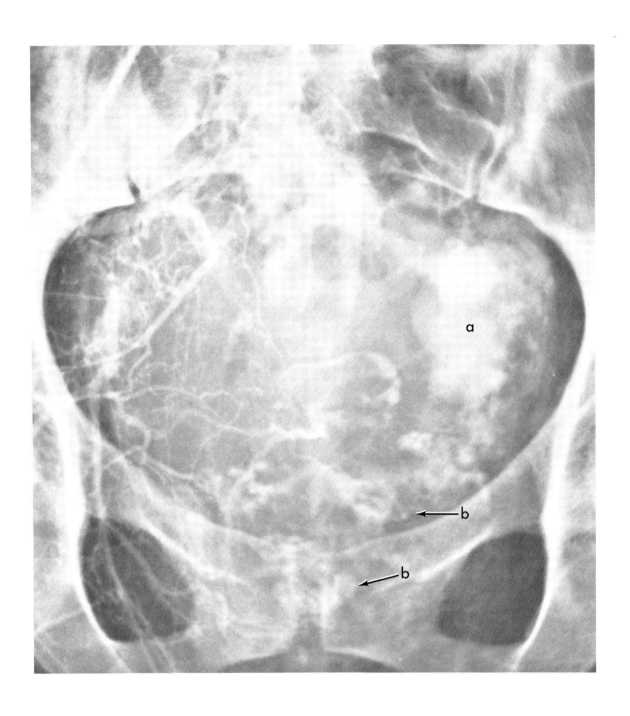

Figure 61 · Choriocarcinoma with Extension / 151

Figure 62.—Choriocarcinoma with subtle vascularity: pelvic angiogram.

Anteroposterior projection: Showing intramural uterine artery branches slightly enlarged and more numerous than normal (**a**). This represented a change from the angiogram obtained six weeks previously and confirmed the presence of active choriocarcinoma.

In July, 1964, the first pregnancy of this patient, age 17, ended in miscarriage. In December she had irregular vaginal bleeding with anemia that required transfusion. In February, 1965, curettage disclosed no chorionic villi. In March there was heavy vaginal bleeding; hemoglobin content was 6.5 g and transfusion was given. HCG excretion was 350 IU/day. Curettings contained trophoblastic elements, possibly choriocarcinoma. Pelvic angiography showed no abnormality, but six weeks later, the angiogram shown here defined invasive trophoblastic neoplasm in the left uterine wall. Chemotherapy was given but the neoplasm progressed. In November hysterectomy disclosed choriocarcinoma in the left side of the uterus. She died of pulmonary and intracranial metastases.

Figure 62, courtesy of Dr. K. D. Bagshawe, Charing Cross and Fulham Hospitals, London.

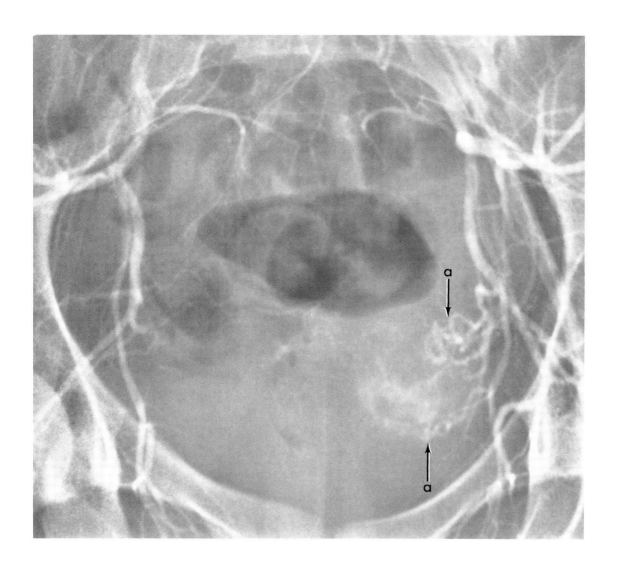

Figure 62 · Choriocarcinoma with Vascularity / 153

Figure 63.—Postmolar choriocarcinoma: pelvic angiograms.

A, early arterial phase, anteroposterior projection: Delineating enlarged uterine arteries (**a**).

B, midarterial phase: Showing dilatation of spiral myometrial arteries (**b**).

(*Continued* on page 156.)

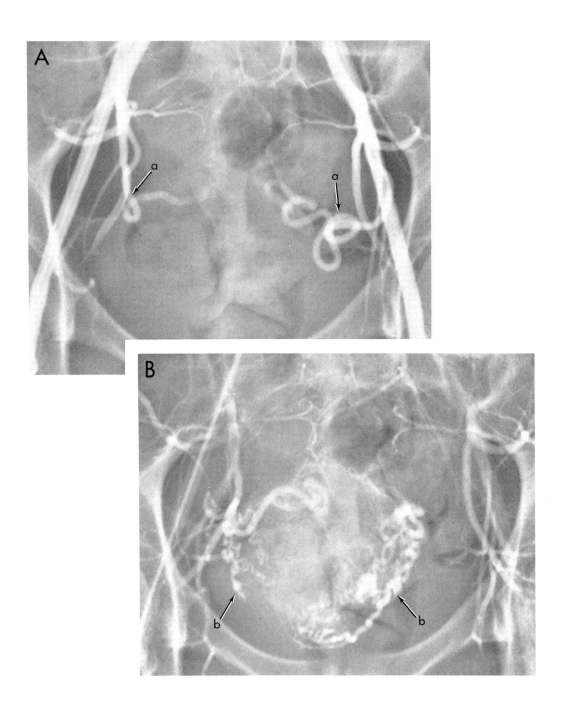

Figure 63 · Postmolar Choriocarcinoma / 155

Figure 63 (**cont.**).—Postmolar choriocarcinoma: pelvic angiograms.

C, arteriovenous phase: Revealing vascular cavities (**c**).

In October, 1964, a hydatidiform mole was evacuated during the first pregnancy of this 22-year-old patient. Menstruation became regular and she was asymptomatic until December, 1965, when heavy vaginal bleeding occurred. She had amenorrhea in February and March, 1966. In May, heavy vaginal blood loss necessitated transfusion of 8 pt. of blood. Curettage revealed no abnormality. Further hemorrhage, headache and hemoptysis followed. In June she was hospitalized with chest pain, weight loss and anorexia. Examination revealed a smooth symmetrical uterine mass the size of a 16 week pregnancy, palpable ovarian cyst and left hemothorax. After four months of treatment with methotrexate and actinomycin D, pelvic angiography was ordered (**A-C**). At hysterectomy the uterine fundus was occupied by a seminecrotic mass of choriocarcinoma. Despite continued chemotherapy, she died of intracranial metastasis.

Comment: The ineffectiveness of chemotherapy is confirmed by the angiographic appearance but must be correlated with HCG assay. On occasion, vascular cavities may persist after successful chemotherapy.

Figure 63, courtesy of Dr. K. D. Bagshawe, Charing Cross and Fulham Hospitals, London.

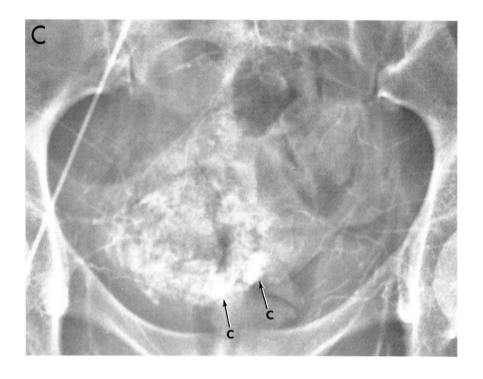

Figure 63 · Postmolar Choriocarcinoma / 157

Figure 64.—Residual or recurrent choriocarcinoma following chemotherapy: pelvic angiogram.

Anteroposterior projection: Showing numerous and enlarged intramural spiral arteries at the site of a residual choriocarcinoma nodule in the uterine fundus (**a**).

Normal term delivery followed this patient's first pregnancy. There was vaginal bleeding in the postpartum period. Pleuritic pain developed and multiple pulmonary nodules were seen in the chest roentgenogram. Curettage revealed choriocarcinoma. During three months of methotrexate and 6-mercaptopurine therapy, a good tumor response was achieved, but HCG elevation indicated relapse two months later. Further chemotherapy was followed by a second relapse. The pelvic angiogram shown here was obtained on the third admission. Subsequent hysterectomy revealed a 1.5 cm nodule of choriocarcinoma in the fundus. Additional chemotherapy followed and she was well four years later.

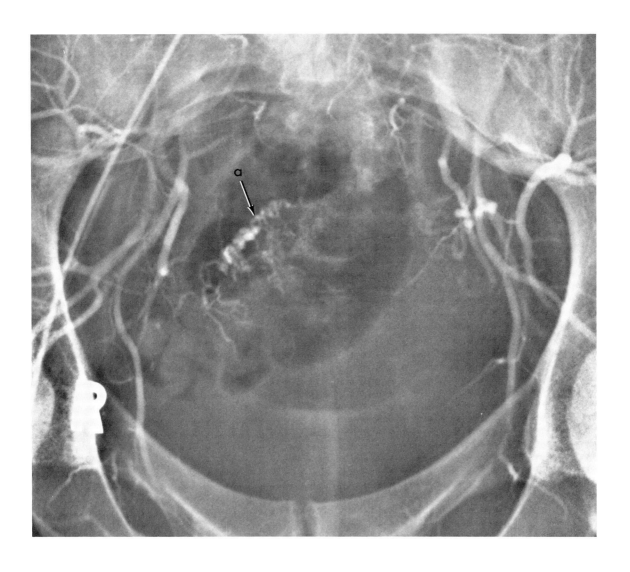

Figure 64 · Choriocarcinoma after Chemotherapy / 159

Figure 65.—Choriocarcinoma persistent in suburethral position after chemotherapy, uterus normal: pelvic angiograms.

A, early arterial phase, anteroposterior view. Internal pudendal branches of the internal iliac arteries (**a**) feed a metastatic choriocarcinoma lesion in suburethral position (**b**).

B, late arterial phase. Intramural vascularity of the left uterine wall suggests persistent small vascular cavity (**c**). No residual tumor was found at this site on pathologic examination, but note the tumor blush in suburethral position (**b**).

A woman, 48, known to have choriocarcinoma had received chemotherapy, but the disease persisted in suburethral position. Angiography was performed preoperatively to assess the presence of other persistent or metastatic disease in the pelvis. The uterus was normal to palpation and no disease was demonstrated elsewhere.

Comment: The persistence of abnormal circulation at the completion of successful chemotherapy has been reported several times. This may explain the vascularity in **B;** however, the suburethral metastasis represented viable tumor.

Figure 65, courtesy of Drs. J. I. Brewer and W. Bundesen, Passavant Hospital, Chicago.

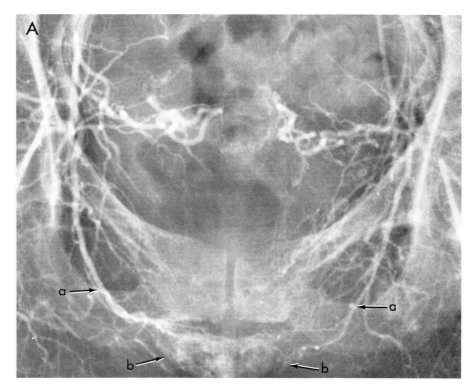

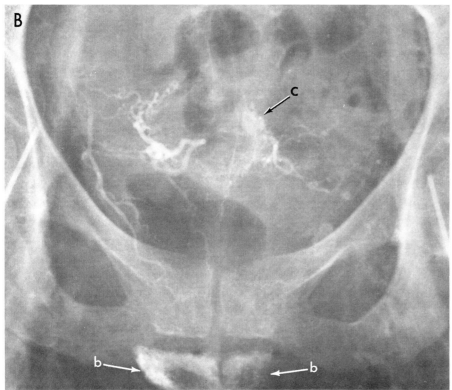

Figure 65 · Choriocarcinoma after Chemotherapy / 161

Figure 66.—Cystosarcoma botryoides of the vagina with extrinsic bladder deformity.

A, plain film, anteroposterior view: Showing soft tissue outline of vaginal tumor (**arrows**). Catheter in bladder.

B, cystogram, lateral view: Revealing extrinsic impression and partial obstruction of the bladder by vaginal tumor (**arrows**).

C, cystogram, oblique projection: Demonstrating bladder deflection without gross invasion (**arrows**).

This 1-year-old girl was noted to have passed hemorrhagic appearing tissue by the vagina.

Figure 66, courtesy of Dr. J. Gwinn, Children's Hospital, Los Angeles.

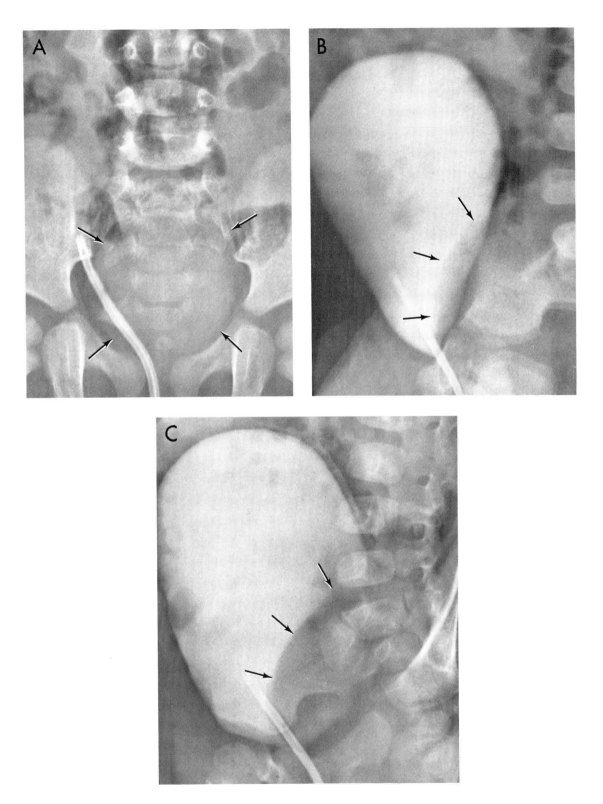

Figure 66 · Cystosarcoma Botryoides / 163

Figure 67.—Cystosarcoma botryoides of the vagina.

A, vaginogram, anteroposterior view: Outlining cystosarcoma botryoides producing multiple polypoid intrusions into the vagina (**arrows**).

B, vaginogram, lateral projection: Delineating tumor protrusion (**arrows**) and distorted vagina.

C, simultaneous excretory urogram and vaginogram, anteroposterior view: Showing bladder (**arrows**) slightly enlarged due to outlet tumor obstruction.

D, 10 months later—barium enema and excretory urogram, anteroposterior view: Demonstrating that the tumor has now invaded the base of the bladder (**arrows**) and displaced the rectum to the left (**a**).

A 2-year-old girl was noted to have vaginal spotting. Vaginography disclosed a polypoid intravaginal mass filling and distorting the vagina. On inspection the tumor was found to involve the cervix and vaginal wall. Surgical resection and 5000 R radiation therapy failed to check the tumor and she died a year after diagnosis.

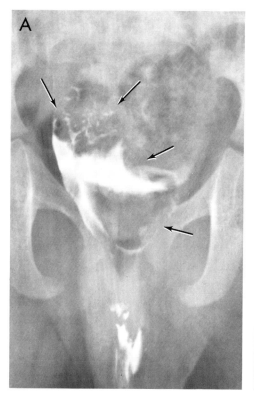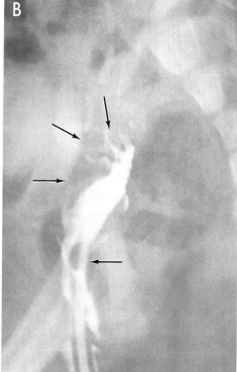

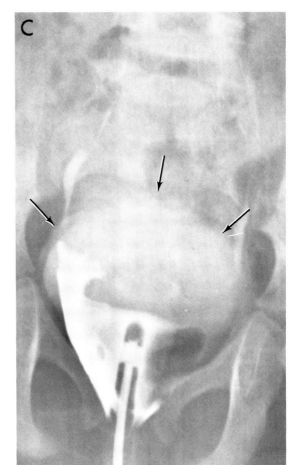

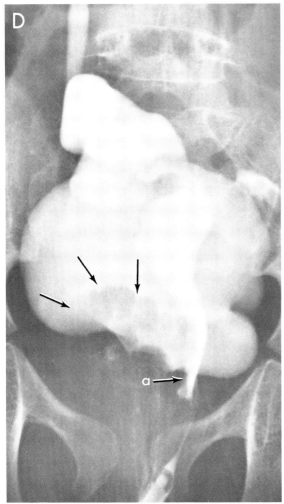

Figure 67 · Cystosarcoma Botryoides / 165

Figure 68.—Cystosarcoma botryoides of the bladder in a male: retrograde cystograms.

A, anteroposterior, and **B,** oblique views: Showing the multilocular character of cystosarcoma botryoides filling the bladder.

A male infant of 18 months had anorexia, abdominal distress and urinary incontinence for about two weeks. An excretory urogram revealed moderate to marked hydronephrosis and hydroureter. A mobile, lobular, lower central pelvic mass was palpable. Suprapubic puncture of the mass failed to produce any urine and only a scanty amount of bloody fluid. Retrograde cystography

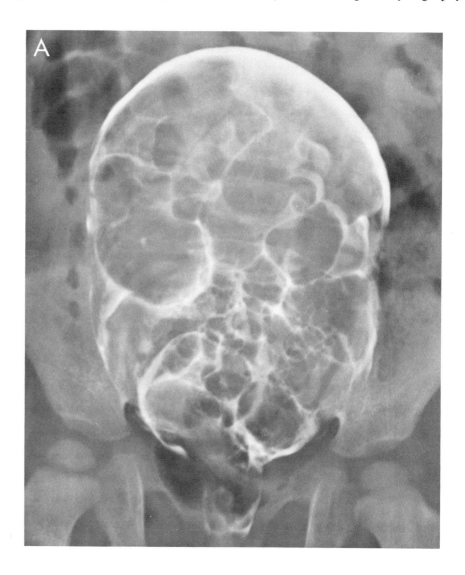

(**A** and **B**) showed the multilocular mass filling the bladder. Cystectomy, prostatectomy and bilateral ureterosigmoidostomy were done, and 18 months later the child was well.

Comment: Strictly speaking, this illustration has no place in this volume since the tumor involves the bladder in a male. However, because cystosarcoma botryoides apparently arises in the mesenchyme of the urogenital ridge and may invade adjacent structures it seems appropriate to illustrate this case which so well demonstrates the gross characteristics of the tumor.

Figure 68, courtesy of Dr. R. C. Brown, Palo Alto-Stanford Hospital, Palo Alto, Calif.

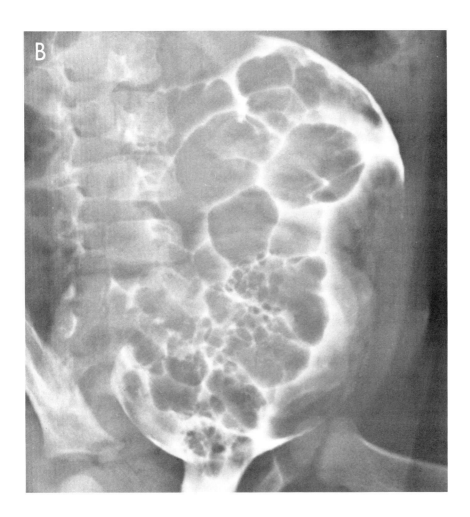

Figure 68 · Cystosarcoma Botryoides in a Male / 167

Figure 69.—Uterine pseudotumors: pregnancy in bicornuate uterus; bifid uterus with hematometra; pelvic pneumograms.

A, posteroanterior view: Revealing bicornuate uterus (**arrows**) with pregnancy in the right horn (**a**) simulating an ovarian neoplasm. Left uterine horn (**b**).

A woman, 27, was seen after having experienced spotting throughout the first trimester of her first pregnancy. Early psychosis and a generally uncooperative attitude made physical examination difficult, but a left ovarian cyst was suspected. As pregnancy progressed the "cyst" seemed to enlarge rapidly, suggesting ovarian neoplasm. Only two films were exposed during pelvic pneumography. A bicornuate uterus was identified to explain the juxtauterine mass. Premature labor occurred at 30 weeks.

B, anteroposterior projection: Demonstrating a bifid uterus (**c**), the left horn of which was palpable, suggesting a left ovarian or adnexal mass.

A girl of 16 described nearly continuous menstrual flow characterized by seven days of heavy flow followed by diminished flow for three weeks. Physical examination was limited by the virginal introitus to one finger. A large mass was suspected in the left pelvis on pelvic examination but was not confirmed on pelvic pneumography. After the bifid uterus was observed, a second cervix was found and dilated. Normal cyclic menses followed.

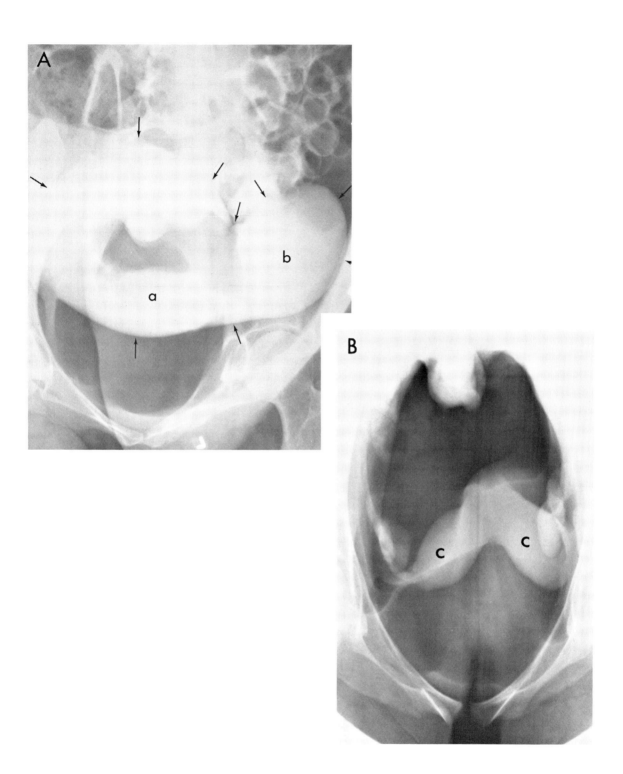

Figure 69 · Pseudotumors / 169

Figure 70.—Adenomyosis of the uterus and endometriosis of the left ovary.

A, pelvic pneumogram, anteroposterior view; **B,** drawing of **A.** The uterus (**a**) is uniformly enlarged. The left ovary is attached to the posterior left side of the uterine fundus and because of adhesions is indistinctly outlined (**b**). Normal right ovary (**c**), sigmoid colon (**d**), bladder (**e**), cecum (**f**).

A gravida V, para 2 woman of 37 complained of menorrhagia, metrorrhagia and increasing dysmenorrhea. Moderately severe premenstrual left lower quadrant pain and bilateral breast lumpiness and tenderness were also described. Five years previously a cesarean section had been performed for abruptio placentae. The left ovary was tender on physical examination. The uterine outline suggested the presence of uterine fibroids. Pelvic pneumography helped to confirm the suspicion of endometriosis and adenomyosis. Surgery revealed an enlarged uterus of normal contour, endometriosis in the left adnexal region with adherence to the left ovary and several tiny endometriotic implants in the right ovary. Adenomyosis of the uterus was established by pathologic examination.

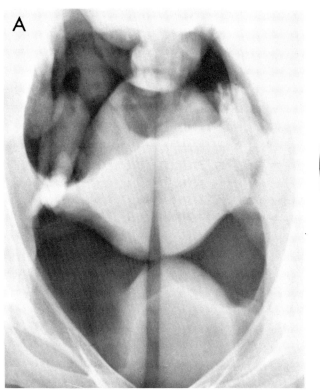
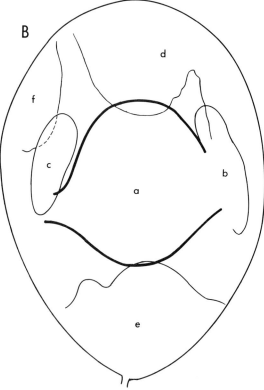

Figure 71.—Pseudotumor produced by an eccentric uterus and cicatrix in the left adnexa.

Pelvic pneumogram, posteroanterior view: Showing the uterus eccentrically positioned to the right of the midline (**a**), creating misleading evidence of a mass on the right. A broad band of cicatrix (**b**) extends from the uterus to left pelvic wall, on top of which lies the left ovary (**c**). The eccentric bladder (**d**) and left adnexal adhesions created a clinical pseudotumor on this side.

While the 43-year-old patient was under treatment for a urethral diverticulum, a pelvic mass was palpated by two examiners, though each placed the mass on different sides of the pelvis. The only symptoms were a "pulling down" sensation and recent menorrhagia. To clarify the uncertainty about the location and origin of the mass, a pelvic pneumogram was ordered. No tumor was demonstrated.

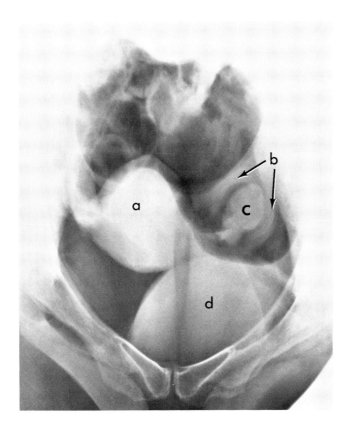

Figure 71 · Pseudotumor / 171

Figure 72.—Pseudotumor—eccentric anatomic variation of the bladder: pelvic pneumograms.

A, posteroanterior projection: Showing the uterus (**a**) situated to the left of the midline, a small subserosal uterine fibroid (**b**), a pseudotumor (eccentric fluid-filled bladder) (**c**), and the ovaries (**d**).

B, same as A, after instillation of air into the bladder (**c**). Broad ligaments (**e**).

A stage I carcinoma of the cervix had been treated four years previously by radium and roentgen therapy. No recurrence was found on subsequent follow-up until the suspicion of pelvic nodules was raised by the patient's internist. Gynecologic consultation and pneumography failed to confirm the presence of metastasis, the eccentric bladder position having initially produced the illusion of an unexplained mass.

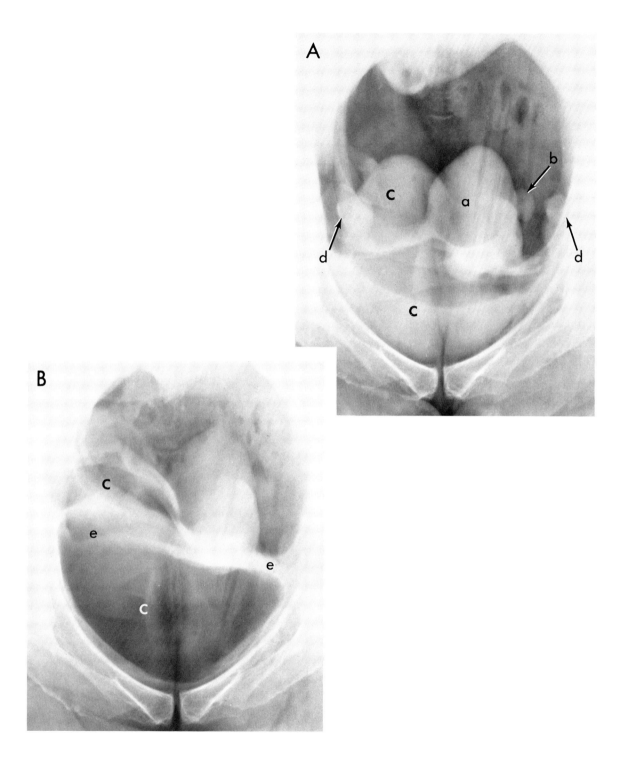

Figure 72 · Pseudotumor / 173

PART 3

The Ovaries and Adnexa

Tumor Characteristics

THE VARIETY and complexity of ovarian tumors not only has made them difficult for the pathologist to identify at times but has even made orderly classification of the entire group the subject of dispute. The more common ovarian tumors and cysts are characterized in the following summary with emphasis on their gross features. No effort has been made to provide a comprehensive description of all recognized entities; such information is available in standard texts.[1-4] Unfortunately there are few radiographic characteristics of ovarian neoplasms or cysts which allow a specific diagnosis and practically none which will allow a confident objective differentiation between benign and malignant tumors. This handicap, however, does not invalidate radiologic investigation in selected cases since there is often a question on physical examination as to whether a mass exists at all. Ovarian enlargements, being difficult to detect and often spontaneously resolving (in the case of nonneoplastic cysts), make routine surgical exploration unacceptable. When clarifying objective information about the presence or type of tumor can be provided by radiologic means, it should be offered.

NONNEOPLASTIC CYSTS OF THE OVARY

NONNEOPLASTIC CYSTS OF THE OVARY.—By far the most common cause of ovarian enlargement is nonneoplastic cysts. Rather than completing the cycle which leads to normal atresia, these cysts persist and grow after graafian follicle rupture. Three principal varieties are recognized; follicular cysts, corpus luteum cysts and theca-lutein cysts.

Follicular cysts may be either single or multiple, are smooth in outline and vary from 2.5–15 cm in diameter. Though they often spontaneously rupture or resolve they may, because of their superficial origin, develop a pedicle, undergo torsion and go on to infarction.

Corpus luteum cysts may become as large as 10–12 cm in diameter and

---

[1] Novak, E. R., and Woodruff, J. D.: *Novak's Gynecologic and Obstetric Pathology: With Clinical and Endocrine Relations* (6th ed.; Philadelphia: W. B. Saunders Company, 1967).

[2] Kraus, F. T.: *Gynecologic Pathology* (St. Louis: C. V. Mosby Company, 1967).

[3] Anderson, W. A. D. (Ed.): *Pathology* (5th ed.; St. Louis: C. V. Mosby Company, 1966), Vol. 2.

[4] Hertig, A. T., and Gore, H.: "Tumors of the Female Sex Organs: Part 3. Tumors of the Ovary and Fallopian Tube," in Armed Forces Institute of Pathology *Atlas of Tumor Pathology*, Sec. IX, Fasc. 33, pt. 3 (1956).

are generally smooth in outline. Hemorrhage occurs in the cyst cavity of some and may cause enlargement and pain in so doing (Fig. 89).

Luteomas of pregnancy (Fig. 86) produced by masses of luteinized cells and polycystic change arise in the ovary under the influence of chorionic gonadotropin. Both ovaries are considerably enlarged during this period of hormonal stimulation, then spontaneously regress after chorionic gonadotropin levels return to normal. Luteomas are particularly common in association with trophoblastic tumors.

STEIN-LEVENTHAL POLYCYSTIC OVARIES.—Bilateral polycystic ovaries associated with Stein-Leventhal disease are characterized by a firm thickened tunica, multiple small follicular cysts which cause ovarian enlargement to one and a half to two times normal, absence of corpora lutea and hyperplasia of the theca interna cells. The ovaries are generally symmetrically enlarged, smooth in outline and oval or lobular in shape (Fig. 92). Clinical features include oligomenorrhea or secondary amenorrhea, anovulation, infertility and hirsutism. Endometrial hyperplasia, presumably due to unopposed estrogen effect, is not uncommonly associated. Because of their consistency and only moderate enlargement, polycystic ovaries in Stein-Leventhal disease are notably difficult to palpate.

ENDOMETRIOSIS.—Endometriosis represents the ectopic or aberrant location of endometrial tissue in the pelvis or, less commonly, the abdominal wall. The most common site of involvement is one or both ovaries, where one may encounter implants only a few millimeters in size up to endometrial cysts as large as 10–12 cm in diameter. Because of their tendency to bleed cyclically, as does normal endometrium, they rupture early and adhesions frequently result between the involved organ and adjacent structures. This may lead to large conglomerate masses comprised of ovaries, uterus, pelvic ligaments and rectosigmoid (Figs. 130–34).

Endometriosis is nearly always seen during active reproductive life and is most common from age 30 to 40. Premenstrual pelvic pain, dysmenorrhea and irregular menses are the most common symptoms. Because of the possibility of management by progestational hormones, objective evidence confirming the clinical diagnosis is most helpful. The same is true, of course, if surgery is being considered.

NEOPLASMS

CYSTADENOMAS.—Cystadenomas may be of mucinous or serous type and together account for over 50% of ovarian neoplasms.[4] Though the two types are of equal frequency and both occur in benign and malignant forms, there are some striking differences.

Serous Cystadenoma and Cystadenocarcinoma.—These tumors range from a few centimeters in diameter to huge tumors filling the pelvis and abdomen, though as a rule they are of moderate size. Typically the benign tumors are inclined to be cystic whereas the malignant ones tend to contain more solid elements. Both externally and internally the surface can be either smooth or studded with papillary growth in either benign or malignant tumors. When present, the papillary growth represents a distinguishing feature of serous tumors as contrasted with the mucinous variety. Though papillary growth does not necessarily imply malignancy, it is a feature which must be viewed with suspicion. Serous tumors can be either uni- or multilocular, are frequently bilateral (estimates range from 20–50%) and are commonly malignant.

One important feature of serous cystadenomas and cystadenocarcinomas is the development of tiny calcified granules which form as the result of degeneration and calcification of tiny papillae (Fig. 85). These are radiographically recognized in approximately 12% of patients.[5] When present, psammoma bodies often cluster in myriads both in the parent tumor and in metastases. Though they occur microscopically in a few other conditions, the radiographic appearance of psammomatous calcification is nearly pathognomonic for cystadenoma and cystadenocarcinoma (Figs. 103, 104, 106–109). A rare exception is shown in Figure 94.

Mucinous Cystadenoma and Cystadenocarcinoma.—Grossly these tumors are generally multilocular and have a smooth exterior surface. Papillary interior growth may occasionally be encountered but is far less common than in the serous tumors. The interior is crossed and compartmentalized by bandlike septa. Most mucinous tumors are of moderate size when detected, but occasionally they are enormous, the world record being 328 lb. Only 5% of mucinous tumors are bilateral. Malignancy is found in only 5% of mucinous tumors, a distinctly lower incidence than in serous tumors.

Calcification in mucinous tumors is uncommon on microscopic examination and is rarely seen radiographically (Fig. 111). Curvilinear calcification which is ascribed to this tumor has generally proved on reassessment to be due to mucinous appendical carcinoma or mucocele resulting in pseudomyxoma peritonei. Despite extensive search for illustrations of such calcification arising in a mucinous ovarian tumor, only one (Fig. 110) could be found, thus attesting to the rarity of this feature.

KRUKENBERG TUMORS.—These tumors are most often bilateral (80%)

[5] Castro, J. R., and Klein, E. W.: The incidence and appearance of roentgenologically visible psammomatous calcification of papillary cystadenocarcinoma of the ovaries, Am. J. Roentgenol. 88:886, 1962.

and metastatic though it is now agreed that they may be primary in the ovary. When metastatic, they most often arise in gastrointestinal primary tumors. Generally, Krukenberg tumors are of moderate size, ovoid or kidney-shaped and nonadherent. No characteristic radiographic features are seen.

GERM CELL TUMORS

DERMOID CYSTS (BENIGN CYSTIC TERATOMAS).—Dermoid cysts (benign cystic teratomas) are of considerable importance and are discussed separately on page 182.

SOLID TERATOMA.—Solid teratoma is a rare tumor which should be considered malignant unless otherwise stated, for only the exceptional case is well-differentiated throughout. All three germ layers provide elements of these tumors, often including the formation of cartilage and bone (Fig. 102) which may be recognized radiographically. They usually appear in children and in young women and when initially found are generally small to moderate in size and commonly adhere to adjacent organs.

DYSGERMINOMA.—Dysgerminoma (Fig. 122) is the female counterpart of male seminoma and in both its clinical course and its response to radiation therapy behaves like seminoma. Two-thirds of patients with this tumor are under 30. The tumors vary greatly in size but are usually well encapsulated. Bilateral tumors are not infrequent, and ascites may be present.

GONADAL STROMAL TUMORS

GRANULOSA AND THECA CELL TUMORS.—Granulosa and theca cell tumors constitute about 10% of solid ovarian tumors and may be seen at any age. Although most behave in a benign fashion, about 25–30% are malignant clinically. Microscopic differentiation between benign and malignant tumors is generally difficult if not impossible. Since these tumors produce estrogen, their most dramatic "feminizing" influences involve prepubertal and postmenopausal patients.

ARRHENOBLASTOMA.—Arrhenoblastoma is most often seen in the age 20–30 group but may be seen any time. Clinical evidence of malignancy is noted in one-fourth to one-third of cases. Depending on the amount of androgen production, varying degrees of defeminization and masculinization appear, sometimes in dramatic form. Arrhenoblastomas are generally small or moderate in size and smooth in outline (Fig. 90).

GONADOBLASTOMA.—This is a rare ovarian tumor but is of relatively greater radiologic importance than its frequency would warrant because of its tendency to calcify. It consists of an intimate mixture of germ cells and elements resembling immature granulosa or Sertoli cells. Cells of Leydig or lutein type are usually present as well. No tumors in this category have been known to metastasize, though they locally invade and contain mitotic figures. They vary in size from a few millimeters to 8 cm. Approximately one-third are bilateral. Scully[6] found that 81% contained microscopic calcification (psammoma bodies), and there is often radiographically visible calcification[7] (Fig. 94).

Gonadoblastoma develops almost exclusively in abnormal gonads. Within the tumor in 50% of cases are areas of overgrowth of germ cell elements which are microscopically indistinguishable from pure dysgerminoma or seminoma. Gonadoblastoma should be considered to be in situ malignancy. The age range is from 1–25 years. Four-fifths of patients with gonadoblastoma are phenotypic females who are commonly virilized.

FALLOPIAN TUBES AND SUPPORTING LIGAMENTS

Inflammatory masses largely consist of obstructive tubal dilatation containing purulent or watery secretion. At times an infected cyst of the ovary may communicate with the lumen of the obstructed tube to form a tubo-ovarian cyst. Although not neoplastic, these masses constitute a much more frequent cause of tubal enlargement than true tumors.

Carcinoma of the fallopian tube is a rare tumor appearing generally in middle age, producing a large sausage-shaped mass and appearing bilaterally in 25% of cases.[1] Unlike pyosalpinx, there are generally no adhesions surrounding the tumor. Rarer still are a variety of benign tumors of the fallopian tube.

Parovarian cysts arising in vestigial remnants of the wolffian body in the mesosalpinx are not uncommon. They are generally oval in shape and of small or moderate size. Fibroid tumors arising in the broad ligament or round ligament are fairly common. The former are usually associated with uterine fibroids and may themselves grow to large size and deflect the uterus from its normal position.

[6] Scully, R. E.: Gonadoblastoma: A review of 74 cases, Cancer 25:1340, 1970.
[7] Cooperman, L. R.; Hamlin, J., and Ng, E.: Gonadoblastoma: A rare ovarian tumor related to dysgerminoma with characteristic roentgen appearance, Radiology 90:322, 1968.

Dermoid Cysts (Benign Cystic Teratomas of the Ovary)

DERMOID CYSTS are benign neoplasms composed of well-differentiated, predominantly ectodermal elements. They comprise 5–10% of cystic neoplasms of the ovary and are frequently (25%) bilateral. Though they are probably congenital, they may appear clinically at any age. While they occur with greatest frequency during reproductive life, nearly 50% of childhood ovarian tumors are dermoid cysts.[1] These cysts vary in size from minute to very large, but 80% are 5–15 cm in diameter and have a smooth oval or round contour.[2]

Of particular importance to the radiologist are locules or cystlike spaces within the tumor containing sebaceous lipoid material which by its greater radiolucency can be detected radiographically. This feature is observed in 36%[3] to 70%.[4] Since these spaces may to varying degrees contain a variety of other germ layer elements and primitive organs, the radiolucency of the mass will vary considerably. One should utilize the more favorable relative absorption characteristics of low kilovoltage exposures to distinguish between fat and water tissue densities.

Of equal importance for radiographic identification is the fact that tooth structures, bone and calcification can be identified within the tumor in approximately 50% of patients.[3,4] The appearance of teeth or bone is typical in nearly one-third of dermoid cysts (Fig. 73–76); in others, though present, these densities cannot be distinguished from other calcific deposits associated with other processes in the pelvis.[3]

The third feature characterizing some dermoid cysts is the so-called capsule, characterized by a thin apparent radiodensity circumscribing the cyst[5,6] (Fig. 80). In reality the encapsulating structure is comprised of skin and a thin layer of attenuated ovarian epithelium. The radiolucent sebaceous mate-

---

[1] Kraus, F. T.: *Gynecologic Pathology* (St. Louis: C. V. Mosby Company, 1967), pp. 367 ff.

[2] Peterson, W. F., *et al.*: Benign cystic teratomas of the ovary: Clinico-statistical study of 1,007 cases with review of the literature, Am. J. Obst. & Gynec. 25:368, 1953.

[3] Sloan, R. D.: Cystic teratoma (dermoid) of the ovary, Radiology 81:847, 1963.

[4] Cusmano, J. V.: Dermoid cysts of the ovary: Roentgen features, Radiology 65:719, 1956.

[5] Robins, S. A., and White, G.: Roentgen diagnosis of dermoid cysts of the ovary in the absence of calcifications, Am. J. Roentgenol. 43:30, 1940.

[6] Good, C. A.: The roentgenologic diagnosis of dermoid cyst of the ovary, Proc. Staff Meet., Mayo Clin. 15:254, 1940.

rial extruded internally delineates the inner aspect of the "capsule," but the explanation of the demarcation of the outer aspect of the capsule is less clear. As judged by specimen radiography in water and vegetable oil with correlative microscopic sections there is insufficient subcutaneous fat in the capsule to delineate its outer surface radiographically. One must speculate that at body temperature, mesenteric fat behaves like a fluid which partially or totally enfolds the dermoid because of the slight negative intra-abdominal pressure. The "capsule" was observed in about 10% of 55 tumors studied by Sloan.[1] In nearly 20%, radiographic evidence of calcification was noted in the peripheral rim of the cyst. Such peripheral eggshell calcification is strongly suggestive of dermoid cyst but may also be seen in uterine fibroids and pelvic arterial aneurysms. Using all radiographic signs in combination, Sloan made a definite diagnosis of dermoid cyst in 40% of lesions.

---

[1] Sloan, R. D.: Cystic teratoma (dermoid) of the ovary, Radiology 81:847, 1963.

Figure 73.—Benign dermoid cyst of the ovary.

A, anteroposterior exposure of the pelvis: Numerous teeth identify the pelvic mass as a dermoid tumor.

B, lateral view: Demonstrating reproductive tract origin of the dermoid tumor.

C, radiograph of surgical specimen: Illustrating bone, teeth and lipoid material in the cyst.

A 12-year-old girl entered the hospital with a brief history of upper abdominal pain and vomiting. Urine examination yielded negative results. The white blood cell count was 10,450, with 90% polymorphonuclear cells. An excretory urogram showed moderate bilateral ureteral compression at the level of the sacral prominences. A 16 cm benign dermoid cyst of the left ovary was removed during surgery. A small dermoid cyst of the right ovary was observed but not removed. Moderate mesenteric adenitis was also seen.

Comment: Dermoid cysts are the commonest pelvic tumors of infancy and childhood.

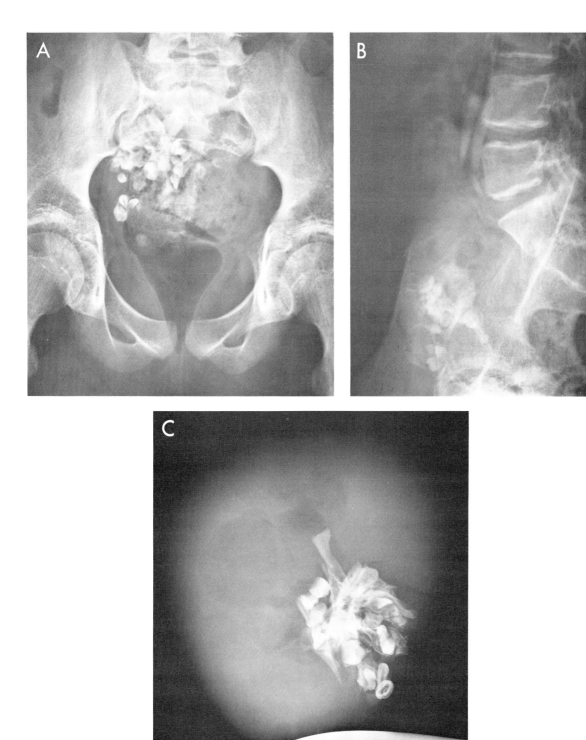

Figure 73 · Benign Dermoid Cyst / 185

Figure 74.—Benign dermoid cyst of the ovary.

A, anteroposterior projection: Showing the radiolucency of a dermoid cyst (**arrows**) but with its dentigerous structure partially obscured by the sacrum. Contrast is seen in the bladder (**a**).

B, oblique projection during excretory urography: Showing the tooth (**b**) to good advantage and peripheral calcification of the cyst wall (**arrows**).

Pelvic pressure symptoms led to excretory urography with disclosure of dermoid cyst of the left ovary.

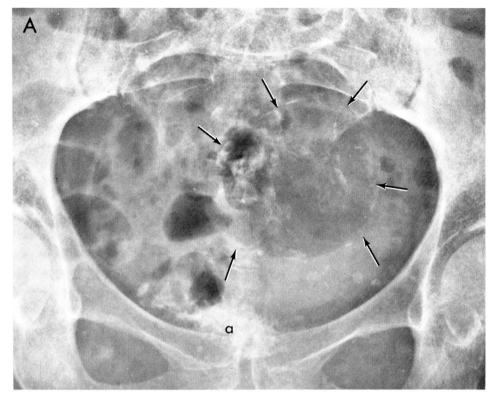

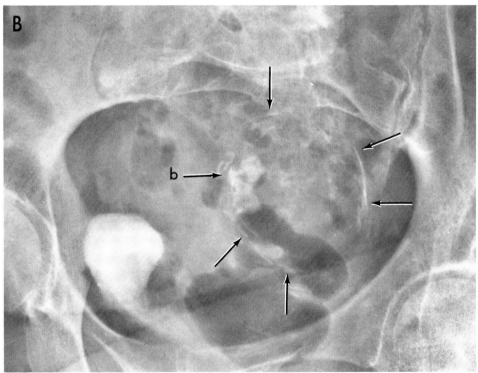

Figure 74 · Benign Dermoid Cyst / 187

Figure 75.—Pedunculated benign dermoid cyst of the ovary.

A, survey film of the abdomen, anteroposterior view: Showing a solitary tooth structure, recognizable only as a spherical density (**a**), associated with a pelvic mass (**arrows**). The moderately distended bladder lies below the dermoid cyst.

B, second exposure, same day as A: Revealing a change of position of the tooth structure (**a**) due to mobility of the pedunculated dermoid. The urine-filled bladder fills the pelvis.

C, radiograph of surgical specimen: Demonstrating clearly the differential density of dermoid content.

A 46-year-old woman had acute lower left quadrant pain, initially thought to be due to sigmoid volvulus. Abdominal exploration revealed bloody peritoneal fluid due to torsion of the pedicle of a large left dermoid cyst with subsequent infarction of the left tube and ovary.

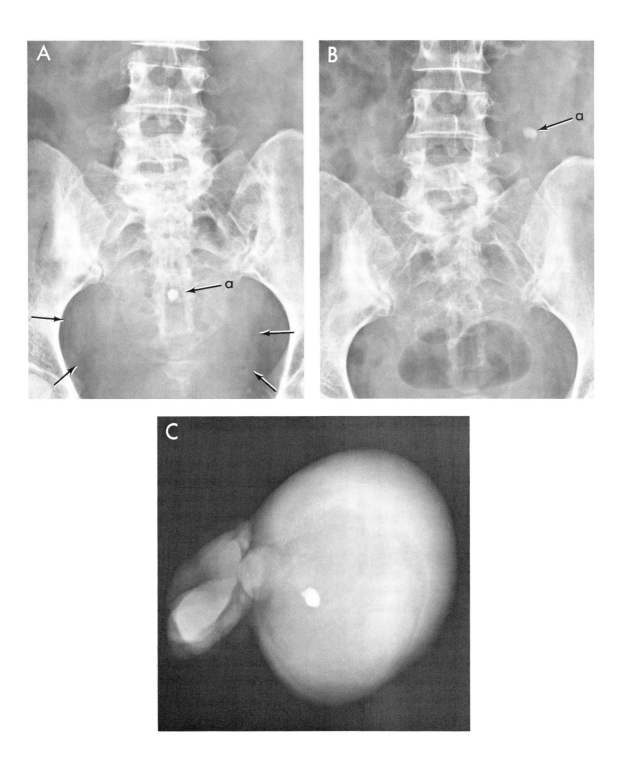

Figure 75 · Pedunculated Dermoid Cyst / 189

Figure 76.—Ovarian dermoid cysts and uterine fibroids.

A, anteroposterior exposure: Revealing coexistent multiple uterine fibroids (**a**) and dermoid cyst of the left ovary (**arrows**). Osseous and tooth structures are contained within the cyst (**b**).

During routine physical examination when the patient was 64, a left lower quadrant mass was palpated. This was believed most likely to represent multiple uterine fibroids, but there was concern about the possibility of an ovarian tumor. Because of psychiatric instability, surgery was not done. She died at age 72 of arteriosclerotic heart disease. The diagnosis of multiple uterine fibroids and left ovarian dermoid was confirmed.

B, anteroposterior view: Disclosing a single tooth providing evidence of a dermoid cyst. Lipoid content of the cyst is difficult to distinguish from intestinal gas.

C, lateral projection: Delineating faint radiolucency surrounding the tooth produced by lipoid cyst content.

This gravida V, para 3 patient of 32 had a firm, mobile mass palpable in the right lower quadrant. Clinical diagnosis was uterine fibroid vs. dermoid cyst. The latter was radiographically confirmed and surgically removed.

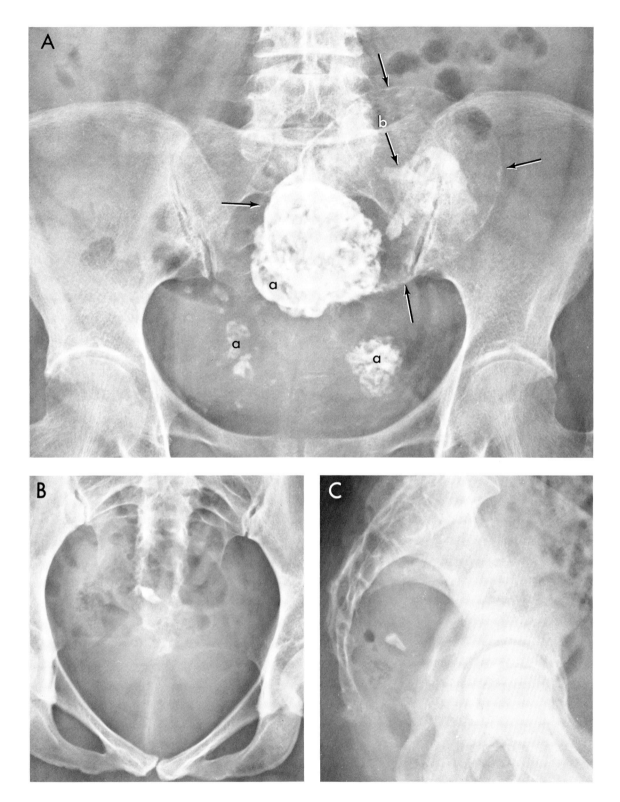

Figure 76 · Dermoid Cysts & Uterine Fibroids / 191

Figure 77.—Dermoid cyst during twin pregnancy and post partum.

A, anteroposterior view: Revealing a dermoid cyst of the right ovary, discovered during the fifth month of a twin pregnancy. Fetal skulls (**arrows**). The dermoid has been markedly displaced up and to the right.

B, same dermoid as in **A,** five months post partum: The lesion has returned to the pelvis.

C, lateral view of **B:** Showing the dermoid in the cul-de-sac of Douglas.

D, radiograph of resected specimen containing teeth, bone and relatively little lipoid material.

A dermoid cyst of the right ovary was discovered during the fifth month of a twin pregnancy (**A**). The patient delivered normally. In the fifth month of a subsequent pregnancy a moderately severe right lower quadrant pain developed, nausea was present and a tender mass could be palpated in the right pelvis. Surgery was performed and the dermoid cyst, now infarcted, was removed (**D**). Pregnancy progressed to normal delivery.

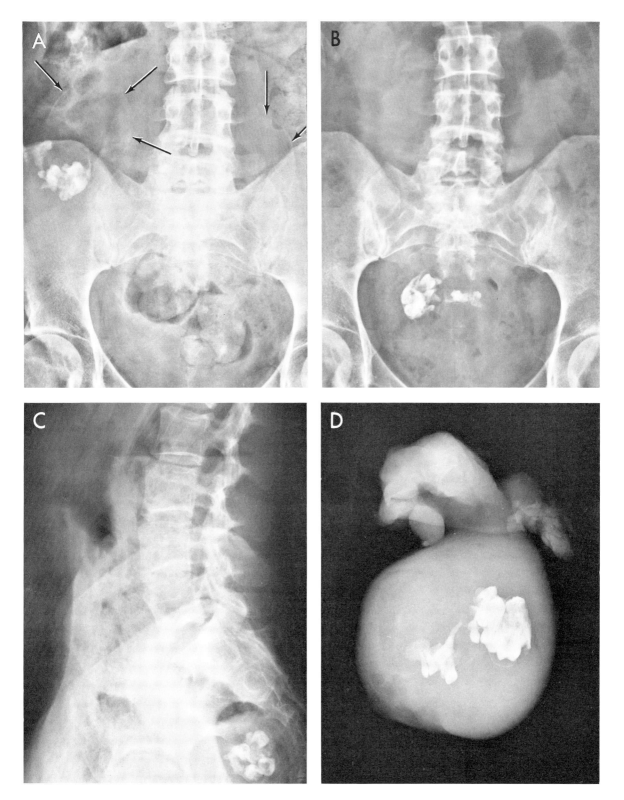

Figure 77 · Dermoid Cyst in Twin Pregnancy / 193

Figure 78.—Benign ovarian dermoid cysts, bilateral and solitary.

A, preliminary film, posteroanterior view: Showing two radiolucent masses (**a, b**), each containing calcific densities.

B, pelvic pneumogram, posteroanterior projection: Demonstrating bilateral ovarian enlargement (**a, b**) corresponding to masses in **A,** confirming the presence of dermoid cysts. Calcifications are barely perceptible (**arrows**). Note the eccentric bladder (**c**), not an uncommon anatomic variant.

During a periodic physical examination this patient of 28 was found to have a slightly enlarged right ovary, believed to be a physiologic cyst. The left ovary was thought to be normal. Surgery nine days after **B** confirmed the presence of bilateral ovarian dermoids.

Comment: Dermoid cysts may vary in fat content. When they largely contain lipoid material their outline may be difficult to perceive against a gaseous contrast, as in the case of the right ovary in **B** (**a**). Dermoids are bilateral in 25% of cases.

C (a second patient), preliminary film, posteroanterior view: Showing dentigerous structure (**d**) surrounded by irregular radiolucency. The latter could be produced by gas or fat. Note the vaginal vault distended by air (**arrows**), with the cervix (**x**) protruding into it.

D, pelvic pneumogram, posteroanterior projection: Revealing a large lobular left ovarian mass (**arrows**) containing dentigerous material superimposed over the uterine outline (**e**) and shifted cephalad by its weight. Additional films demonstrated the anatomic detail more completely, and a normal right ovary. Diagnosis was ovarian dermoid.

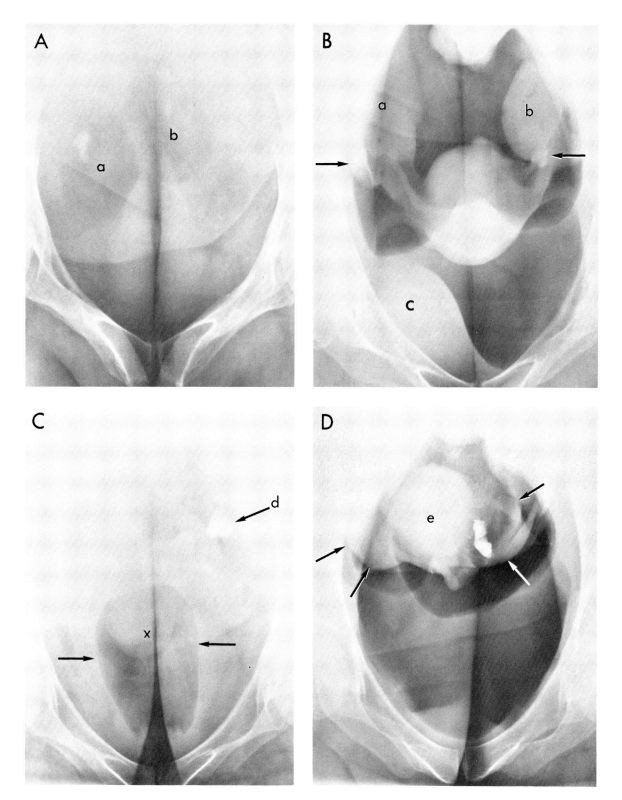

Figure 78 · Benign Dermoid Cysts / 195

Figure 79.—Benign dermoid cyst of the ovary.

A, preliminary film, posteroanterior projection: Revealing an ovarian dermoid. Note teeth (**a**) and surrounding fat density (**b**).

B, pelvic pneumogram, posteroanterior projection: Delineating the size and contour of the right ovarian dermoid (**c**). Normal uterus (**d**) and left ovary (**e**).

C, pelvic pneumogram, right anterior oblique projection: Showing the dermoid cyst of the right ovary (**c**); uterus (**d**); left ovary (**e**).

In this patient an enlarged right ovary was palpated on routine bimanual examination during care for erosion of the cervix. A typical dermoid cyst was removed during surgery.

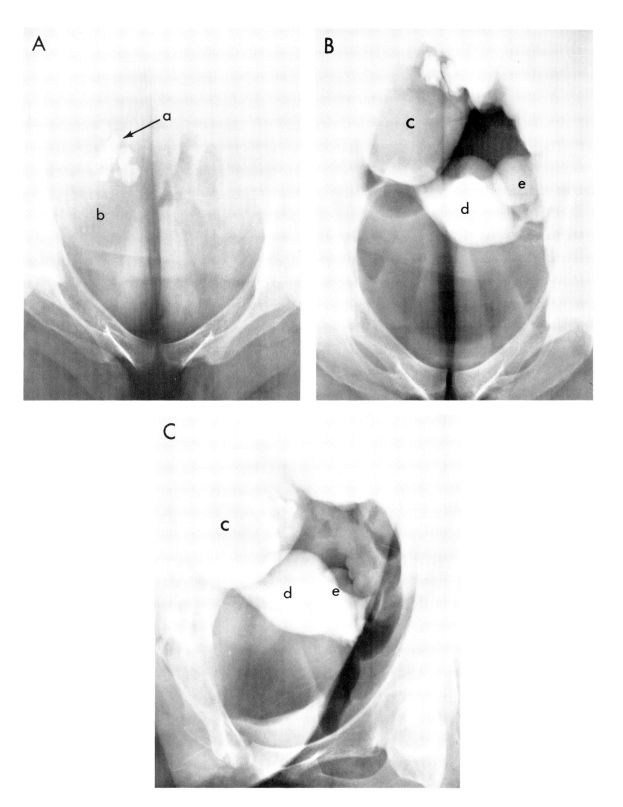

Figure 79 · Benign Dermoid Cyst / 197

Figure 80.—Large benign dermoid cyst of the ovary: "capsule" sign.

A, preliminary film, posteroanterior view: Clearly demonstrating a radiolucent mass, the periphery of which is distinctly seen (**arrows**; see text, p. 182, for explanation). The mass contains dentigerous structure (**a**).

B, pelvic pneumogram, posteroanterior exposure: Delineating a large left ovarian mass (**arrows**), right ovary (**b**) and uterus (**c**).

C, pelvic pneumogram, left lateral decubitus projection: Showing size and outline of dermoid (**arrows**) somewhat better.

On premarital examination a large rubbery pelvic mass, suspected to be a dermoid cyst, was palpated. Surgery confirmed the clinical and radiologic diagnosis and a 12 cm mass was removed.

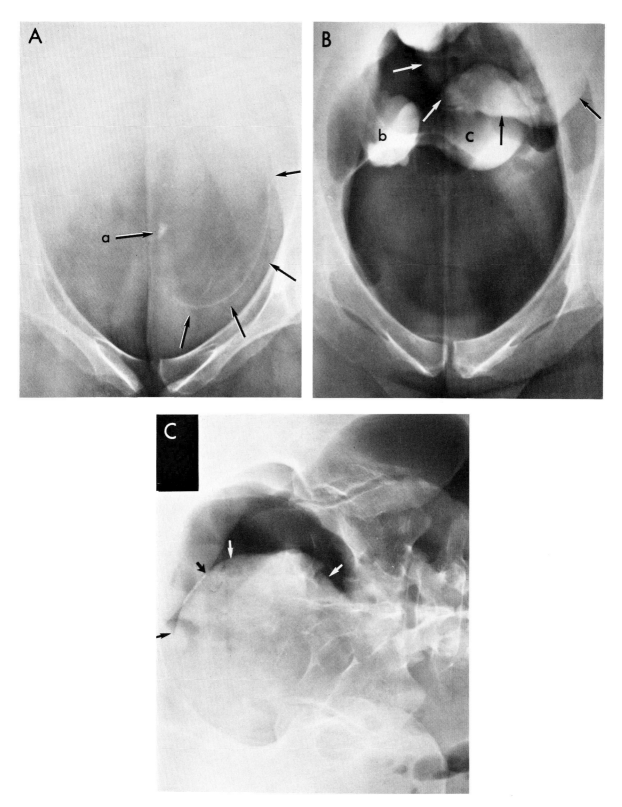

Figure 80 · Dermoid Cyst: "Capsule" Sign / 199

Figure 81.—Benign ovarian dermoid cysts; one case with uterine fibroids.

A, pelvic pneumogram, posteroanterior view, and **B,** drawing of **A:** Showing pedunculated right ovarian dermoid (**a**) containing calcifications (**arrows**), kidney bean-shaped pedunculated uterine fibroid (**b**), small subserous fibroid (**c**) and slightly enlarged uterus containing intramural fibroids (**d**). Urinary bladder (**e**); sigmoid colon (**f**).

In this 37-year-old gravida I patient a tender soft mass was palpable in the right adnexa. She had a history of surgery at age 16 with removal of a left dermoid cyst and left salpingo-oophorectomy. The pneumographic findings shown here were confirmed at surgery.

C, pelvic pneumogram, posteroanterior projection: Showing a large, relatively radiolucent right ovarian mass (**arrows**) containing calcification or ossification and a slightly cystic left ovary (**g**). Uterus (**h**).

This asymptomatic 40-year-old patient came for her first physical examination in 15 years. Diagnosis was ovarian cyst vs. third-degree retroverted uterine fundus. Subsequent surgery disclosed a 10 cm right ovarian benign dermoid cyst and a tiny corpus luteum cyst of the left ovary.

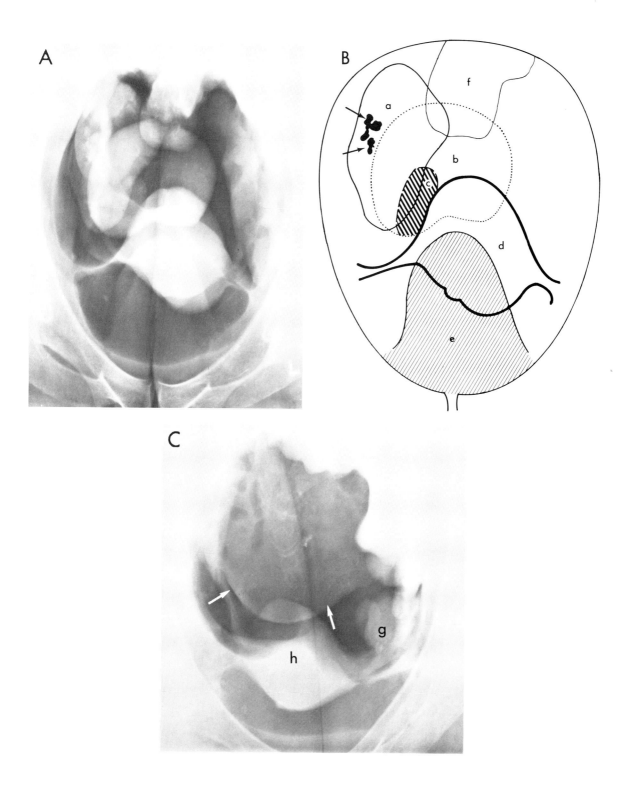

Figure 81 · Dermoid Cysts: Uterine Fibroids / 201

Figure 82.—Benign dermoid cysts of the ovary.

A, anteroposterior projection: Showing central radiolucency, partial peripheral "radiopaque" rim (**arrows**) and the dental structure within, which characterize the left ovarian dermoid cyst.

B, radiograph of the surgical specimen after it was opened.

Acute onset of central pelvic pain with accompanying slight temperature elevation and leukocytosis in this patient of 41 led to clinical and radiologic diagnosis of dermoid cyst. At surgery a multiloculated, benign, partially infarcted dermoid cyst of the left ovary was removed.

Comment: The appearance of dentigerous structure in the right pelvis suggests right ovarian dermoid also, but the surgical record did not describe one. Perhaps the surgeon was preoccupied by the infarcted left dermoid cyst.

C, pelvic pneumogram, posteroanterior projection: Demonstrating a right ovarian dermoid cyst containing tooth structure (**a**). Lipoid content is difficult to appreciate when surrounded by gas. Round ligament (**b**); uterus (**c**); left ovary (**d**).

A mass had been inconsistently palpated in the right lower quadrant over a four year period in this 27-year-old patient. Menses were normal and no symptoms were described. Subsequent surgery confirmed the radiologic diagnosis of dermoid cyst.

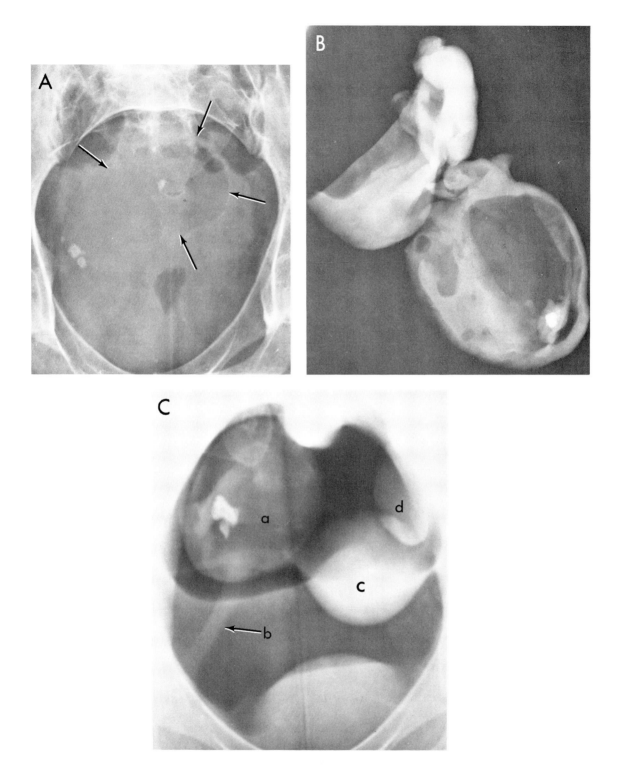

Figure 82 · Benign Dermoid Cysts / 203

Figure 83.—Pseudomucinous cystadenoma of the ovary.

A, preliminary film, anteroposterior view: Illustrating a large pelvic-abdominal mass (**arrows**) which blends with the outline of the urinary bladder (**x**).

B, barium enema (postevacuation film), anteroposterior view: Revealing extrinsic displacement of the colon and terminal ileum by the large right ovarian tumor.

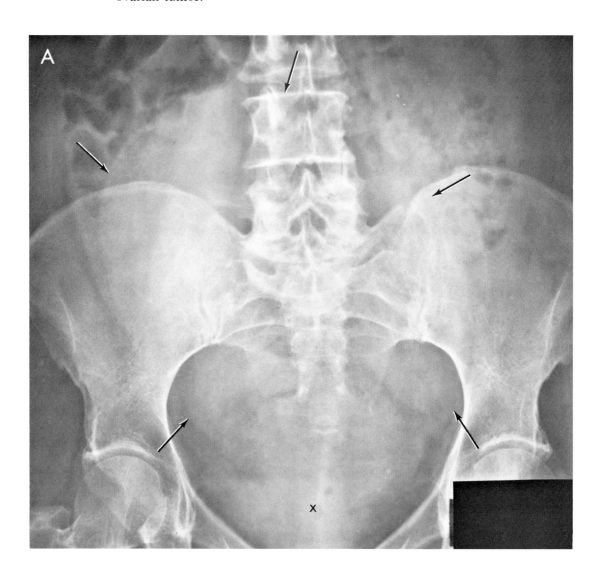

Abdominal distention and urinary frequency brought this 65-year-old patient to her physician. Long-standing interstitial cystitis had previously caused similar symptoms, but on this occasion a large central pelvic mass reaching nearly to the umbilicus was palpated and abdominal films were ordered. A mucinous cystadenoma of the left ovary, measuring 14 cm in diameter, was discovered and a total hysterectomy performed.

Comment: Such a large tumor may obscure anatomic relationships, invalidating the usefulness of pelvic pneumography except for visualizing the peritoneal surfaces for implants. Surgery is obviously necessary.

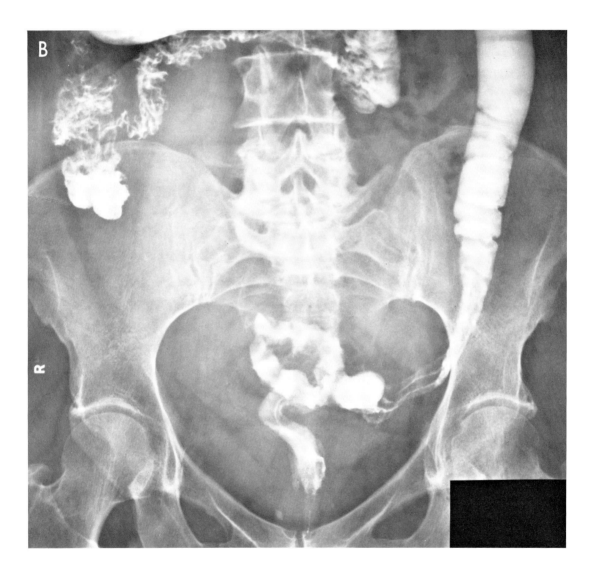

Figure 83 · Pseudomucinous Cystadenoma / 205

Figure 84.—Mucinous cystadenoma of the ovary.

A, preliminary film, anteroposterior view: Showing a homogeneous rounded mass (**a**) filling the pelvis. Separation from the bladder is manifested by extravesical fat (**b**). The sigmoid colon is elevated.

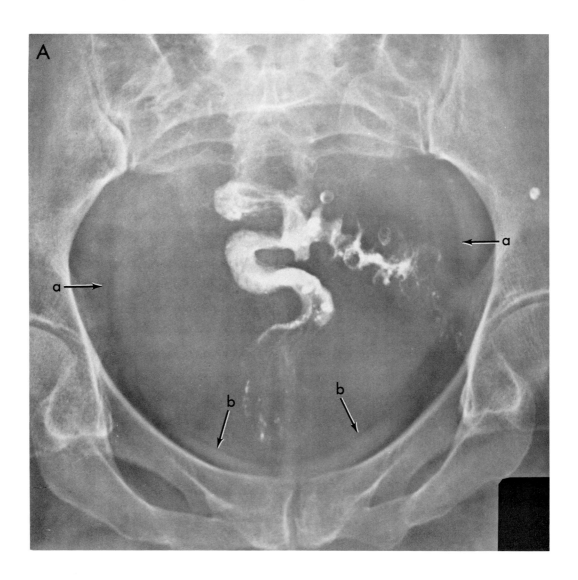

B, excretory urogram: Delineating extrinsic pressure on the bladder dome confirmed by contrast in the bladder (**x**).

A woman of 74 had noted abdominal swelling for a year and occasional rectal bleeding for the past two to three months. Sigmoidoscopic examination revealed narrowing of the upper sigmoid and blood coming from above this point. A cystic mass believed to be ovarian was easily palpated in the pelvis. It proved to be an 18 × 14 × 10 cm mucinous cystadenoma of the right ovary.

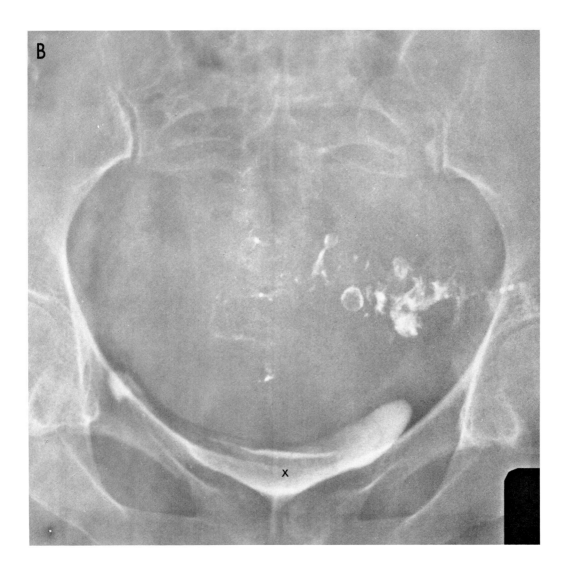

Figure 84 · Mucinous Cystadenoma / 207

Figure 85.—Benign papillary serous cystadenoma of the ovary.

A, preliminary film, anteroposterior view: Showing widely scattered small aggregates of calcification (**x**) in a large pelvic mass (**arrows**). Such calcification generally indicates calcified psammoma bodies in serous adenomas of the ovary.

B, barium enema, posteroanterior view (prone position): Revealing extrinsic pressure of a pelvic mass on the colon and terminal ileum.

C, pelvic pneumogram, right anterior oblique projection: Demonstrating the large smooth-bordered mass (**arrows**) which arises from the partially atrophic left ovary (**a**). Uterus (**b**); right ovary (**c**).

D, pelvic pneumogram, left anterior oblique projection: Showing normal right ovary (**c**), uterus (**b**) and peritoneal surfaces free from implants.

Abdominal protuberance and pressure symptoms were the chief complaints of this patient of 52. A large soft mass was palpable and was suspected to be a lipoma in the abdominal wall. The radiographic studies were conducted to delineate the size, origin and type of tumor if possible.

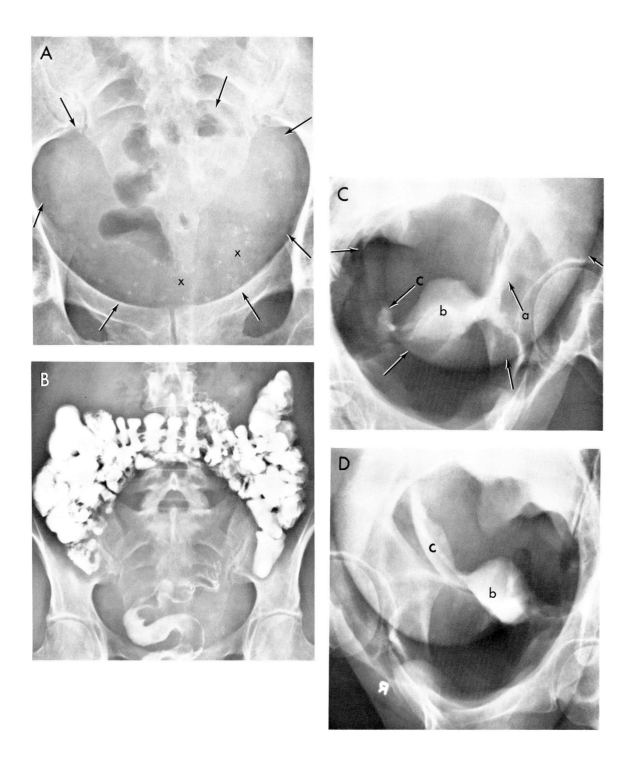

Figure 85 · Benign Serous Cystadenoma / 209

Figure 86.—Large ovarian cyst accompanying pregnancy.

Anteroposterior exposure: Demonstrating a pregnant uterus containing a fetal skeleton (**x**) and a right ovarian cyst (**arrows**).

A 19-year-old primigravida entered the hospital complaining of vaginal bleeding. Her last normal menstrual period had occurred 7½ months before. Some vaginal bleeding had also occurred for a 10 day interval during the second month of pregnancy. No fetal life was perceptible at the time of admission. The result of a frog test for pregnancy was reported to be negative. The initial abdominal film showed no sign of a fetal skeleton (apparently due to fetal motion), but a repeat film 1 week later (shown here) delineated skeletal structure in the left upper abdomen. At surgery a right ovarian cyst which was nearly as large as the pregnant uterus was encountered. The cyst was removed and recovery was uneventful.

Comment: Theca-lutein cysts of one or both ovaries occasionally occur in conjunction with normal pregnancy. They are commonly seen in patients with hydatidiform mole or choriocarcinoma and sometimes reach very large size.

Figure 86, courtesy of Dr. J. J. McCort, Valley Medical Center, San Jose, Calif.

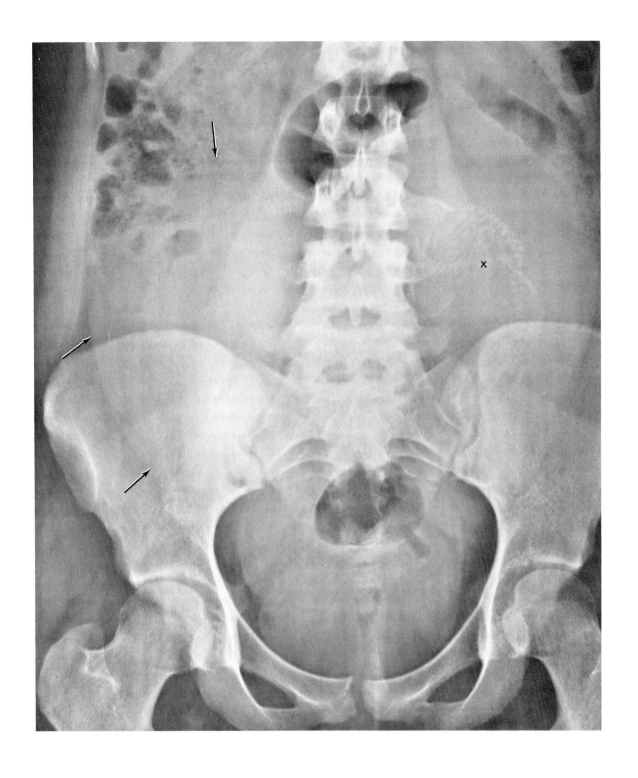

Figure 86 · Ovarian Cyst in Pregnancy / 211

Figure 87.—Pedunculated hydatid cyst of the ovary.

A, pelvic pneumogram with central beam angled 20° caudad, postero-anterior exposure: Showing hydatid cyst (**a**), right ovary (**b**), uterus (**c**) and slightly cystic left ovary (**d**).

B, similar exposure with central beam angled 10° caudad: Showing the entirety of the right ovarian hydatid cyst (**a**), right ovary (**b**), uterus (**c**) and left ovary (**d**).

A woman of 20 who had missed two menstrual periods was examined and a right ectopic pregnancy was suspected. Menstruation then occurred. The mass remained intermittently palpable. At surgery an 8 × 10 cm hydatid cyst attached by a short pedicle to the right ovary was found.

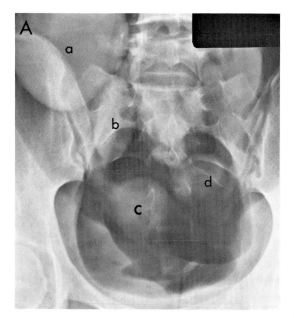

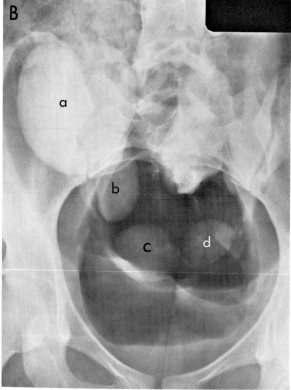

Figure 88.—Cyst of a remaining ovary.

Pelvic pneumogram, posteroanterior projection: Revealing a large smooth-bordered mass (**a**) arising from the remaining right ovary. The uterus and left ovary had been removed at surgery.

A gravida III, para 3 patient of 35 had had hysterectomy and unilateral oophorectomy 10 years previously. Records of the surgery could not be obtained. Slight pain in the right lower quadrant was present. On pelvic examination a mass believed to be the right ovary was detected. It was thought to be an ovarian cyst on pelvic pneumography. On clinical follow-up the mass had disappeared.

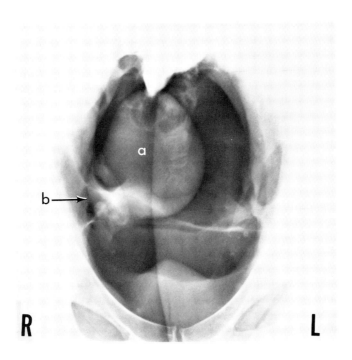

Figure 88 · Cyst of a Remaining Ovary / 213

Figure 89.—Hemorrhagic corpus luteum cyst.

A, pelvic pneumogram, posteroanterior projection: Delineating a sausage-shaped left adnexal mass (**a**). It is not clear whether the mass is of ovarian or tubal origin.

B, combined pelvic pneumogram and uterosalpingogram, posteroanterior exposure: Demonstrating a normal left tube and identifying the mass (**arrows**) as the left ovary. Round ligaments (**b**).

A 24-year-old woman complained of chronic menstrual irregularity and recent cramping pain in the lower left quadrant. Dyspareunia was also present. Presumptive diagnosis was pelvic inflammatory disease or endometriosis, for which she was treated during the next 18 months. During this time, pelvic examinations by three gynecologists and one urologist revealed no abnormality. The pelvic studies shown here were made because of persistent unexplained pain. The left ovarian mass was found to be a hemorrhagic corpus luteum cyst, and its surgical removal eliminated the long-standing pain.

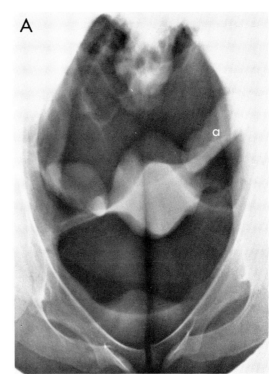

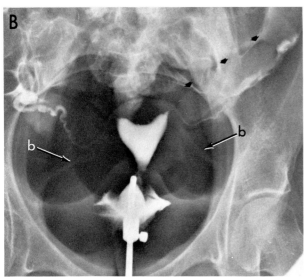

Figure 89 · Hemorrhagic Corpus Luteum Cyst / 215

Figure 90.—Arrhenoblastoma.

A, pelvic pneumogram, posteroanterior projection: Disclosing an enlarged left ovary (**a**) which is incompletely seen, and the uterus (**b**) displaced to the left. Adhesions (**c**) extend to the sigmoid. Normal right ovary (**d**).

B, pelvic pneumogram, with tube angled 10° caudad, left anterior oblique projection: Showing the left ovarian tumor (**a**) to better advantage. Uterus (**b**); right ovary (**d**).

A girl of 12½ years had a history of amenorrhea, hirsutism and masculinization. Heavy menstrual flow initially followed menarche at age 10; the flow gradually tapered off over the next two years, followed by amenorrhea. A somewhat masculine voice and muscle volume and distribution were observed. No clitoral enlargement was present. The 17-ketosteroid and 17-hydroxycorticosteroid levels were at the upper limits of normal. The gynecologist suspected a masculinizing ovarian tumor, but because of the virginal introitus a satisfactory bimanual examination was not possible. No estrogen effect was seen on cervical cytology. The sella turcica was normal. Pelvic pneumography confirmed the presence of a left ovarian mass, and during surgery this was identified as an arrhenoblastoma. Following surgery all masculinizing features disappeared and normal menstruation ensued.

Figure 90, from Stevens, G. M.: Radiol. Clin. North America 5:87, 1967.

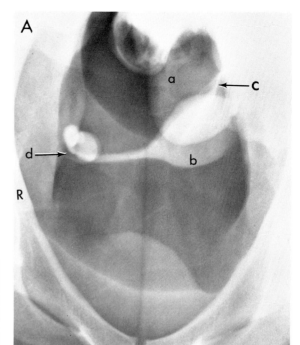

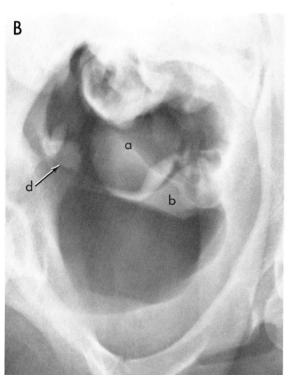

Figure 90 · Arrhenoblastoma / 217

Figure 91.—Serous cyst of the ovary.

Pelvic pneumogram, posteroanterior projection: Showing a moderate-size, smooth-bordered right ovarian mass (**a**) and normal uterus (**b**) and left ovary (**c**). Sigmoid colon (**d**).

Because of midcycle bleeding this gravida 0 patient, age 22, sought gynecologic consultation. A history of increasing hirsutism, acne and menstrual irregularity was obtained. On initial pelvic examination the findings were normal, but subsequently a right adnexal mass was suspected. The pelvic pneumogram confirmed the presence of a right ovarian mass. A 6 × 6 × 5 cm serous cyst of the right ovary was removed during surgery. The following year the patient had a normal pregnancy and delivery.

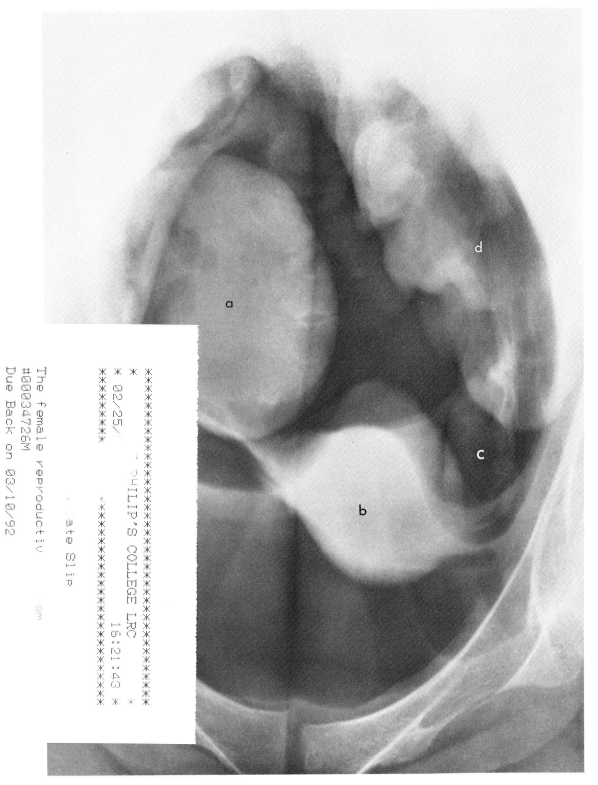

Figure 91 · Serous Cyst / 219

Figure 92.—Stein-Leventhal syndrome with polycystic ovarian enlargement.

Pelvic pneumogram, posteroanterior projection: Revealing the right and left ovaries (**a**) to be symmetrically enlarged, with a smooth, oval contour, and disproportionately large in relation to the uterus (**b**). There is no sign of adhesions or implants suggesting endometriosis, considered to be a clinical possibility. Fluid-filled cecum (**c**); sigmoid colon (**d**).

A gravida 0 patient of 24 complained of dysmenorrhea and spotting. Menstruation had been grossly irregular from age 17 and recent cycles were anovulatory. Moderate hirsutism was present. The right ovary was palpably enlarged, but the left was thought to be normal. Both Stein-Leventhal syndrome and endometriosis were considered to be clinical possibilities. Surgery with bilateral wedge resections of Stein-Leventhal ovaries resulted in ovulatory cycles and pregnancy.

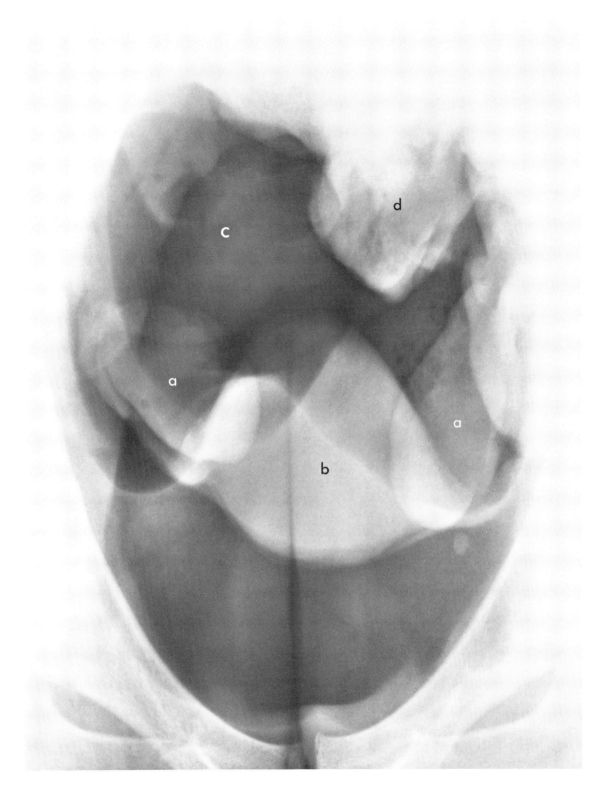

Figure 92 · Stein-Leventhal Syndrome / 221

Figure 93.—Bilateral Brenner tumors.

A, pelvic pneumogram, with central ray angled 10° caudad, postero-anterior projection: Showing a large, smooth-bordered right ovarian mass (**a**). The posterior margin of the mass is not delineated. The left ovary (**b**) is slightly enlarged, the uterus (**c**) normal.

B, pelvic pneumogram, with central ray angled perpendicular to the floor: Demonstrating the posterior border of the right ovarian tumor to better advantage (**a**), and the left ovary containing a small tumor (**b**). Uterus (**c**).

A 30-year-old unmarried woman complained that about 18 months earlier the interval between menstrual cycles had diminished to two weeks. A slow, 17 lb. weight gain and gradually increasing hirsutism were additional complaints. Physical examination disclosed a masculine escutcheon, normal clitoris and firm, enlarged right ovary. Adherence to a prescribed diet resulted in loss of 30 lb. and normal menstrual periods for a year. Thereafter the menstrual cycle lengthened, flow became scanty and hirsutism increased. The right ovary remained enlarged, mobile and firm. The uterus and left ovary were believed to be normal. Pelvic pneumography confirmed the presence of a smooth-bordered right ovarian mass and slightly enlarged left ovary. At surgery an 8 × 6 × 4.5 cm Brenner tumor was removed on the right and a similar but much smaller one from the left ovary. Thereafter menstruation was normal.

Comment: Brenner tumors generally occur in women past 50. Though nearly always benign, rare examples of malignancy have been reported. Between 5 and 10% of the patients exhibit some estrogenic effect (*Novak's Textbook of Gynecology* [6th ed.; Baltimore: Williams & Wilkins Company, 1961].)

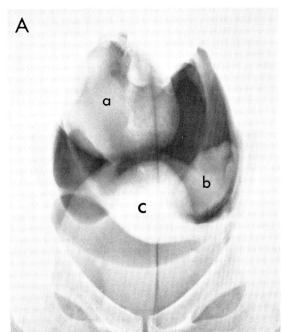

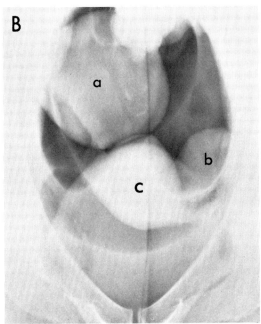

Figure 93 · Bilateral Brenner Tumors / 223

Figure 94.—Bilateral gonadoblastoma.

A, preliminary film, anteroposterior view: Illustrating bilateral ovoid calcified masses (**a**), the left being larger than the right.

B, pelvic pneumogram, posteroanterior projection: Demonstrating that the calcifications seen in **A** are ovarian. The uterus (**b**) is situated eccentrically to the right.

A nulliparous patient of 18 had attained physical maturation by age 15½, with normal hair development and stature, but had never menstruated. Breast size diminished from 32-C to 32-A after age 15½, and a minimal estrogen effect was noted on cervical cytology. A normal family history was obtained.

Radiographic examination of the pelvis disclosed bilaterally calcified ovaries. Bilateral oophorectomy led to identification of bilateral gonadoblastomas.

Comment: Gonadoblastoma is a rare but radiographically significant benign neoplasm occurring most often in abnormal gonads of chromatin-negative phenotypic females who are commonly virilized. Psammoma calcification is generally present and often visible radiographically.

Figure 94, courtesy of Dr. V. Voakes, Menlo Park, Calif.; and Cooperman, L. R., *et al.:* Radiology 90:322, 1968.

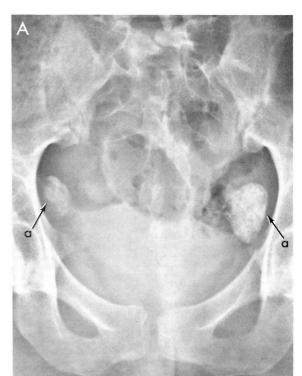

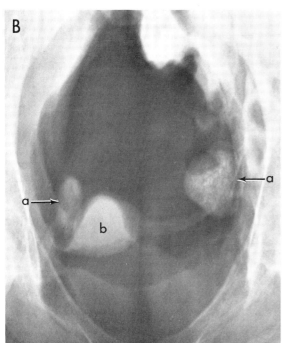

Figure 94 · Bilateral Gonadoblastoma / 225

Figure 95.—Pseudomucinous cystadenoma: pelvic arteriograms.

A, early arterial phase, anteroposterior projection: Showing the uterine arteries (**4**), with the right much larger than the left; superior rectal artery (**9**); right ovarian artery (**10**), and adnexal branches from the right uterine artery (**11**). The tumor is large and occupies the central and right side of the pelvis. The uterine position in the left pelvis is identified by the uterine arteries.

B, late arterial phase: demonstrating uterine arteries (**4**), right ovarian artery (**10**) and anastomoses with adnexal branches (**11**).

C, later phase: Delineating ovarian artery (**10**), adnexal tributaries (**11**) and tumor vessels (**arrows**) extending into the solid mass. The cystic portion is in the central pelvis.

A woman, age 36, had had irregular vaginal bleeding for four months and increasing abdominal girth. A mass was palpable to the level of the umbilicus. A large, essentially cystic pseudomucinous cystadenoma was identified at surgery.

Figure 95, courtesy of Drs. C. Rådberg and I. Wickbom, Gothenberg, Sweden.

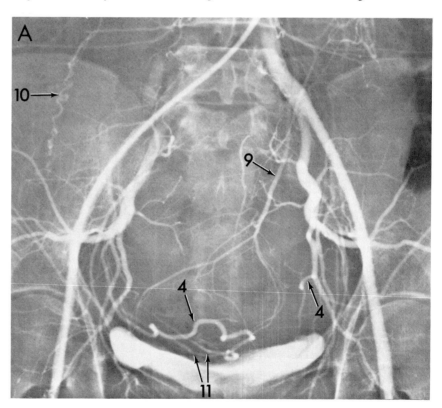

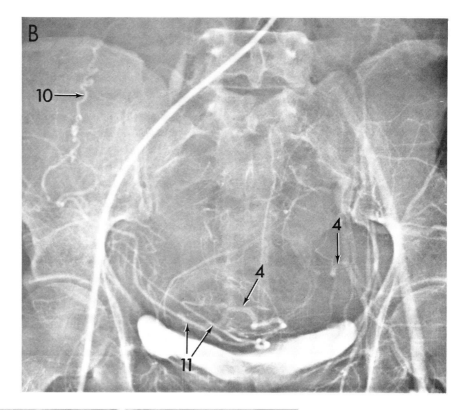

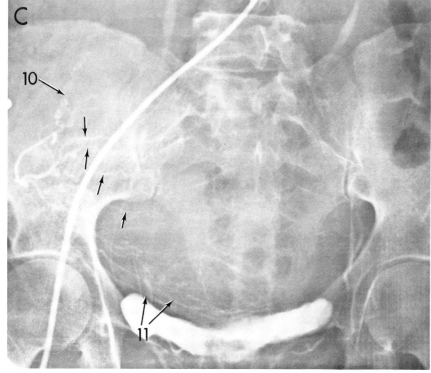

Figure 95 · Pseudomucinous Cystadenoma / 227

Figure 96.—Bilateral ovarian fibromas and right parovarian cyst.

A, pelvic arteriogram, arterial phase, anteroposterior view: Showing the uterine arteries (**4**), with hypervascularity seen at **a** produced by the end-on view of the marginal branches of these arteries and a retroflexed uterus.

B, pelvic arteriogram, late arterial and capillary phase: Showing the uterus opacified in the central pelvis. Enlarged adnexal branches of the uterine arteries are seen (**b**) with small tumor vessels (**c**) arising from the adnexal branches.

C, pelvic pneumogram, posteroanterior projection: Clearly demonstrating the bilateral ovarian enlargement (**d**). A parovarian cyst (**e**) seen on the right is not identified in the arteriograms. Uterus (**f**).

A woman of 45 was seen because of irregular vaginal bleeding and a movable mass to the left of the uterus. Clinical diagnosis was pedunculated uterine fibroid vs. an ovarian mass. Bilateral ovarian fibromas and a right parovarian cyst were found at surgery.

Comment: Although bilateral adnexal masses can be seen in the arteriograms, the vasculature does not distinguish between a benign and a malignant process. The greater clarity of the margins of the ovarian tumors in the pelvic pneumogram is apparent.

Figure 96, courtesy of Drs. C. Rådberg and I. Wickbom, Gothenberg, Sweden.

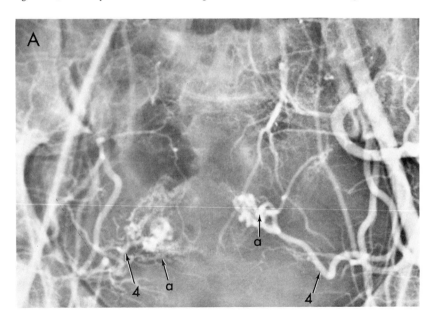

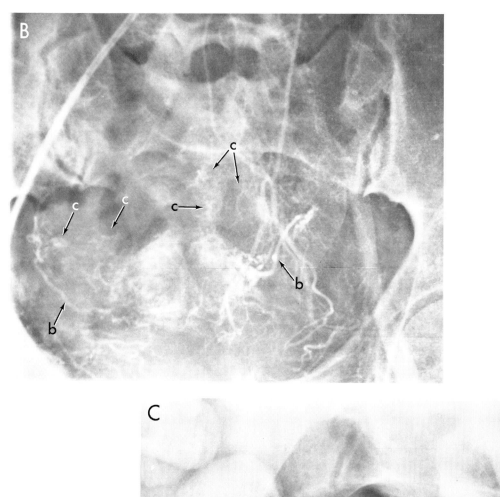

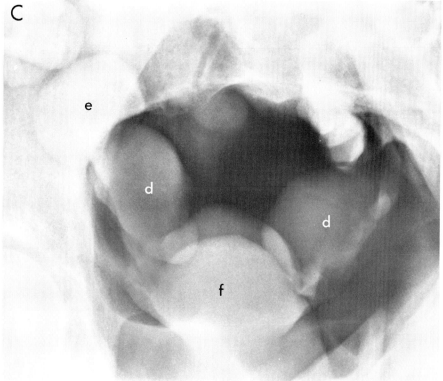

Figure 96 · Bilateral Fibromas & Parovarian Cyst / 229

Figure 97.—Corpus luteum of pregnancy simulating ovarian neoplasm: pelvic arteriograms.

A, early arterial phase, anteroposterior projection: Delineating the uterine arteries (**4**), the right being larger than the left. Superior rectal artery (**9**).

B, late arterial phase: Demonstrating the enlarged uterus (**a**), the right side of which is more richly vascularized due to placental sinusoids; a highly vascularized corpus luteum of pregnancy in the left ovary (**b**), and residual contrast in the superior rectal arteries (**9**).

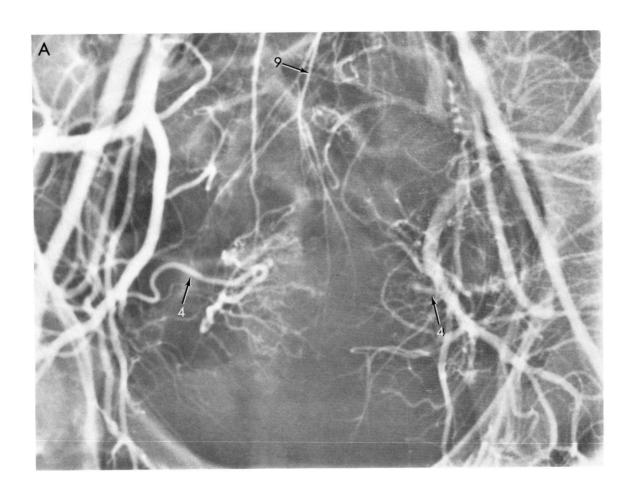

A patient of 21 had her last menstrual period seven weeks before being seen. Pain had been present in the left lower abdomen for two weeks. The uterus was large and soft, and a tender mass was palpable in the left adnexal region. Ectopic pregnancy?

Comment: Corpus luteum of pregnancy can simulate both ovarian neoplasm and salpingitis. The placental opacification differentiates in this case, however.

Figure 97, courtesy of Drs. C. Rådberg and I. Wickbom, Gothenberg, Sweden.

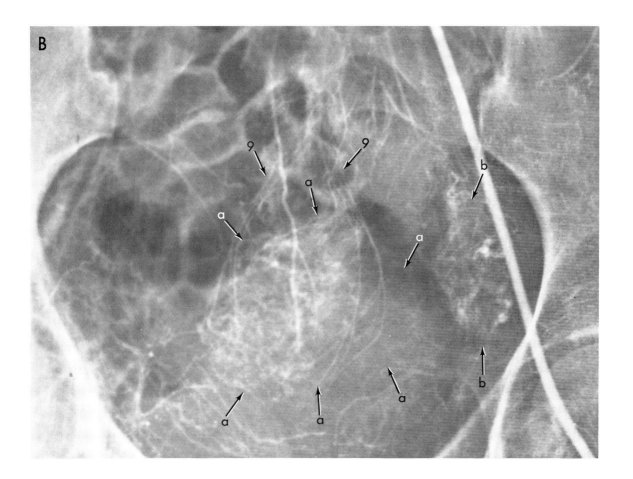

Figure 97 · Corpus Luteum of Pregnancy / 231

Figure 98.—Unilateral inflammatory mass—salpingitis: pelvic arteriograms.

A, early arterial phase, anteroposterior view: Delineating normal uterine arteries (**4**), superior rectal artery (**9**) and enlarged adnexal branch of the right uterine artery (**11**).

B, late arterial phase: Showing residual contrast in the adnexal branch of the right uterine artery (**11**) and numerous arterial tributaries to the inflammatory mass caused by salpingitis (**arrows**).

A woman, age 47, had had irregular vaginal bleeding since her last normal menstruation eight months previously. Erythrocyte sedimentation rate was 65. An irregular right posterior uterine mass was palpated. The clinical diagnosis was ovarian neoplasm vs. uterine fibroid.

Figure 98, courtesy of Drs. C. Rådberg and I. Wickbom, Gothenberg, Sweden.

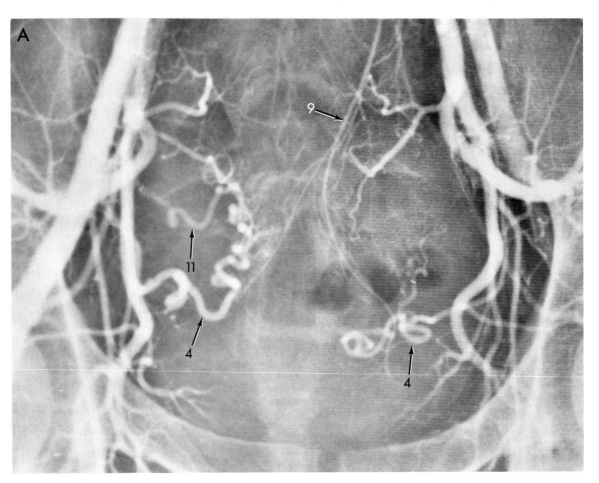

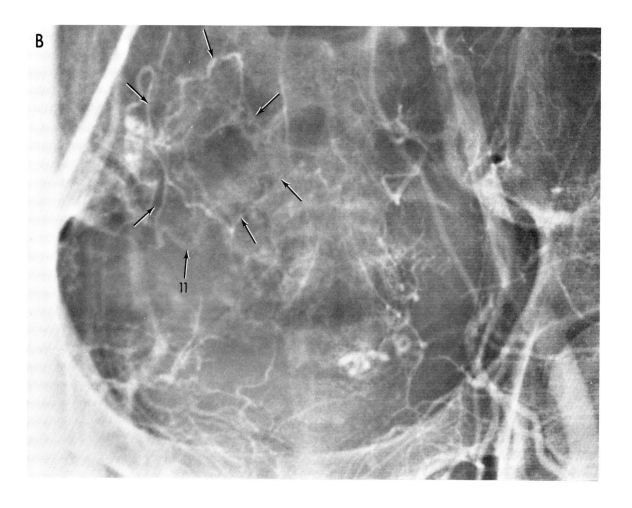

B

11

Figure 98 · Unilateral Salpingitis / 233

Figure 99.—Bilateral salpingitis.

A, pelvic arteriogram, late arterial phase, anteroposterior view; and **B,** drawing of **A:** Delineating the uterus (**a**) and adnexal branches of the uterine artery enlarged on both sides, producing a plexus of abnormal vessels (**b**) extending to the bilateral salpingitis.

The patient, age 20, had had her last normal menstrual period six weeks before, with scant vaginal bleeding at two week intervals thereafter. A mass was palpated to the left of the uterus, suspected to be an ectopic pregnancy.

Figure 99, courtesy of Drs. C. Rådberg and I. Wickbom, Gothenberg, Sweden.

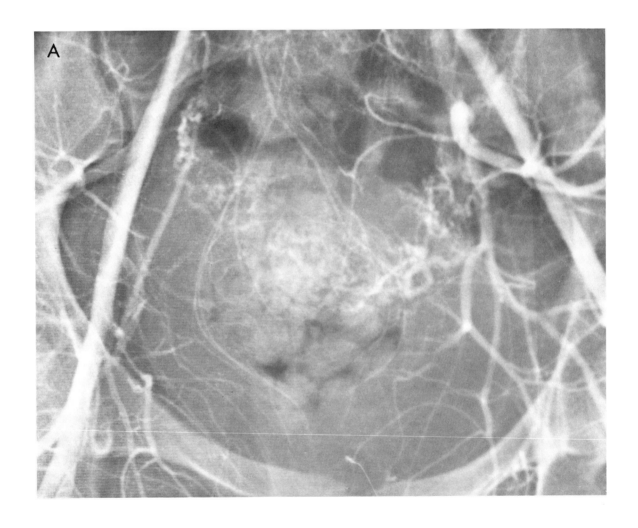

B

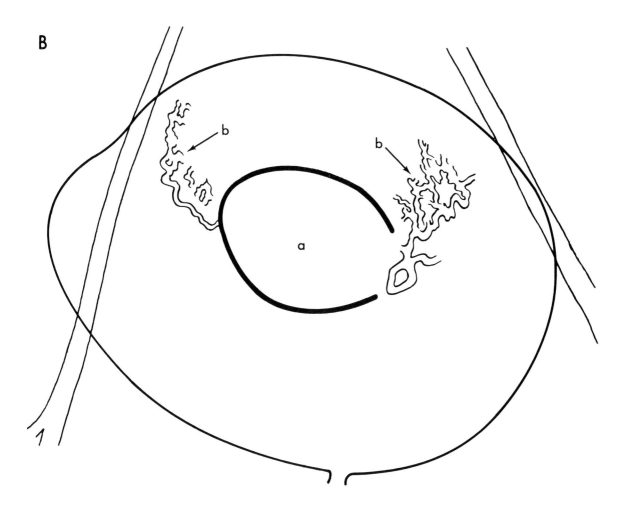

Figure 99 · Bilateral Salpingitis / 235

Figure 100.—Papillary cystadenocarcinoma with ascites.

A, excretory urogram, anteroposterior view: Showing a large pelvic mass deflecting the ureters. Voluminous ascites produces a homogeneous density in the abdomen.

(*Continued* on page 238).

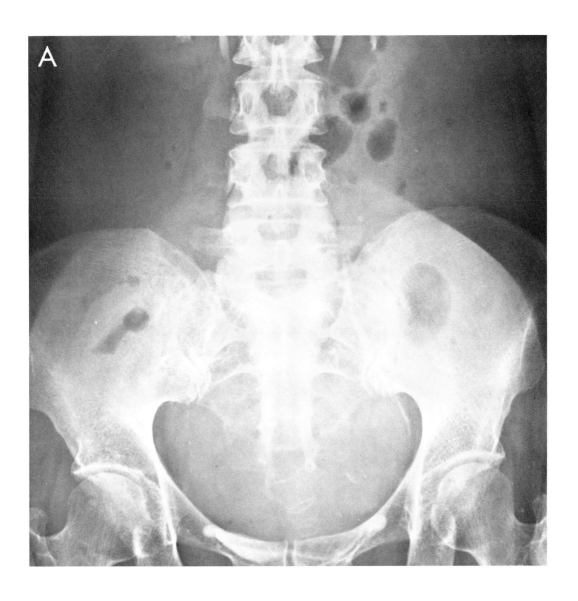

A

Figure 100 · Papillary Cystadenocarcinoma / 237

Figure 100 (cont.).—Papillary cystadenocarcinoma with ascites.

B, postevacuation of barium enema, anteroposterior view: Revealing central position of colon and terminal ileum and homogeneous abdominal density characteristic of massive ascites. Note difference from appearance of the large ovarian cyst in Figure 83.

C, lateral exposure during barium enema: Indicating pressure on the barium-filled rectum and sigmoid by the tumor and ascites.

A woman, 69, complained of increasing girth and progressive constipation, nausea and pelvic pressure for two months. A hard pelvic mass arising in the pelvis and extending into the right lower quadrant was palpable. Ascites was suspected. Surgical exploration revealed a large amount of free peritoneal fluid, widespread metastasis and a large papillary cystadenocarcinoma arising from the right ovary. Radiation therapy (1700 rad tumor dose in nine weeks), intraperitoneal nitrogen mustard and testosterone were not effective and she died five months after surgery.

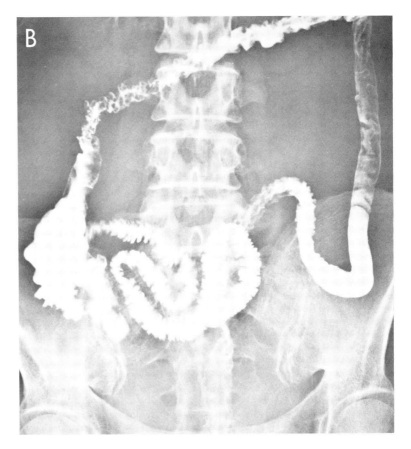

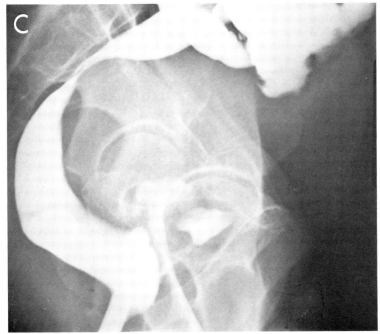

Figure 100 · Papillary Cystadenocarcinoma / 239

Figure 101.—Papillary adenocarcinoma.

A, preliminary film, anteroposterior projection: Showing pelvic mass (**arrows**) separated from the bladder (**a**). The right flank outline is distinct (**b**). No intraperitoneal fluid is evident.

B, same projection as **A,** during excretory urography: Revealing separation of pelvic tumor from the bladder and uterine compression of the right side of the bladder. Ascites in the cul-de-sac could produce a similar picture, except for the appearance in **C.**

C, barium enema, posteroanterior view: Demonstrating extrinsic sigmoid colon displacement distinguishing the pelvic mass from fluid.

This woman of 55 had carcinoma of the cervix treated by radium 15 years previously. Her chief complaint now was severe sudden left flank and lower quadrant pain, with slight dysuria, frequency and black stools for 2 days. A movable left pelvic and flank mass was palpated. At surgery a

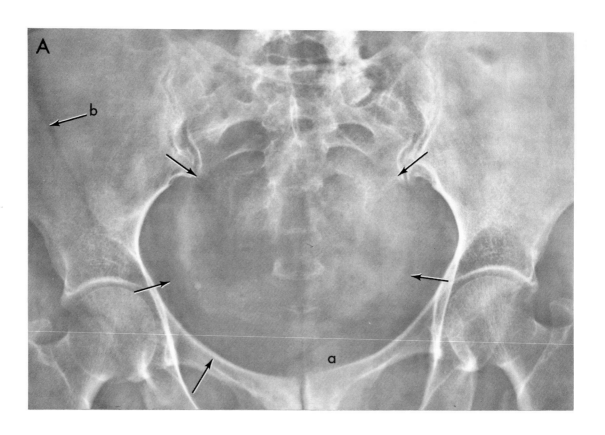

moderately differentiated papillary adenocarcinoma of the left ovary with extension into the sigmoid mesentery was found; hysterectomy and bilateral salpingo-oophorectomy were performed. A 4000 rad pelvic tumor dose was given. She died 20 months after the tumor was discovered.

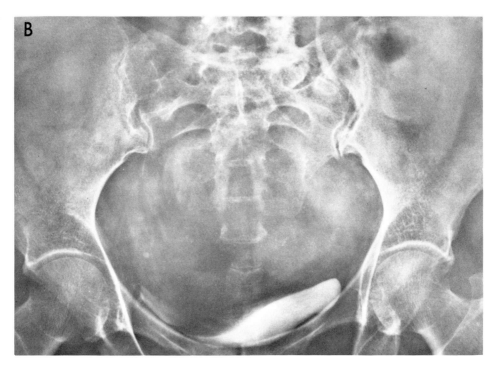

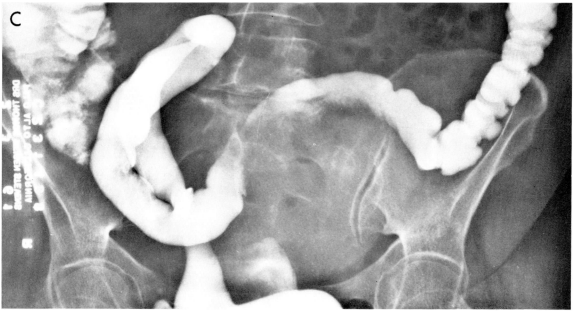

Figure 101 · Papillary Adenocarcinoma / 241

Figure 102.—Malignant teratoma of the ovary.

Anteroposterior exposure during intravenous urography: Revealing a large, smooth-bordered pelvic and abdominal mass. In the upper pole a network of calcific strands is present (**arrows**). Low-grade pyelocalyceal dilatation is produced by extrinsic compression of the ureters. There is metastatic partial destruction of the right pedicle of the second lumbar segment (**x**).

A 33-year-old woman had a three month history of enlarging abdomen and pelvic mass and right leg pain. The colon was extrinsically displaced by the mass. Mild bilateral hydronephrosis due to ureteral compression was demonstrated. At operation a 2600 g left ovarian tumor was encountered. The capsule was smooth and glistening. No papillary excrescences were seen, and only one adhesion at the upper pole of the mass was identified. No abdominal metastases were seen. Microscopically the tumor proved to be a malignant teratoma with islands of calcified hyaline cartilage, and bone.

Figure 102, courtesy of Dr. J. J. McCort, Valley Medical Center, San Jose, Calif.

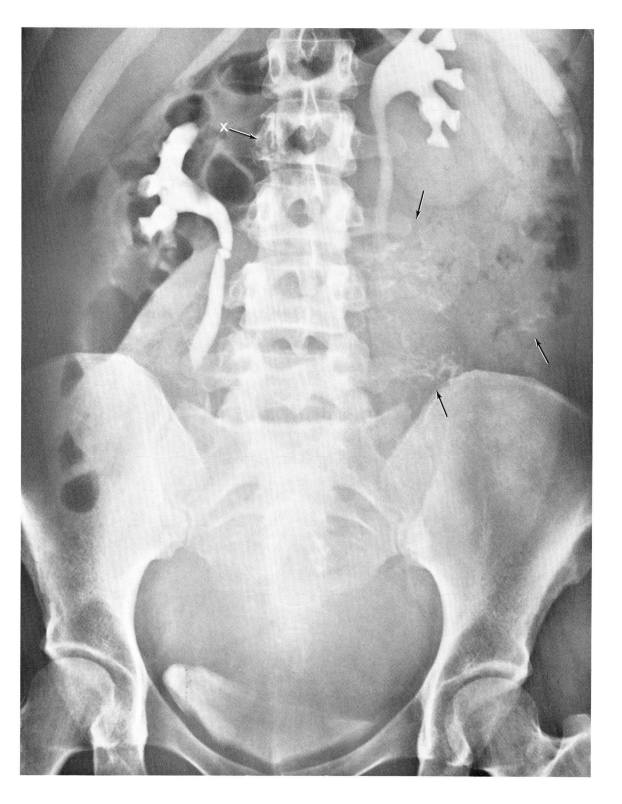

Figure 102 · **Malignant Teratoma** / **243**

Figure 103.—Papillary adenocarcinoma with psammomatous calcification.

A, plain film, anteroposterior view: Revealing amorphous masses of psammomatous calcification in the pelvic component (**x**) of a papillary adenocarcinoma of the ovary. Note metastatic calcified tumors in the liver and left upper quadrant (**arrows**).

B, anteroposterior barium enema study: Delineating an area of sigmoid narrowing produced by the ovarian neoplasm (**arrow**). Psammomatous

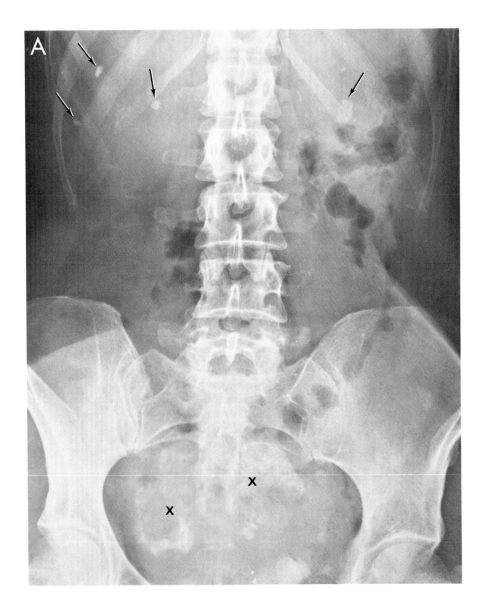

calcification is sometimes confused with residual barium. When seen simultaneously the difference in density is clear.

The patient, age 58, experienced an acute intestinal obstruction, for which surgical exploration was done. Papillary adenocarcinoma of the ovary with widespread mesenteric involvement was found. A cecostomy was performed. Postoperatively, 3300 rads was given to the pelvic midplane, with good palliation for about 18 months. She died 20 months after the tumor was discovered.

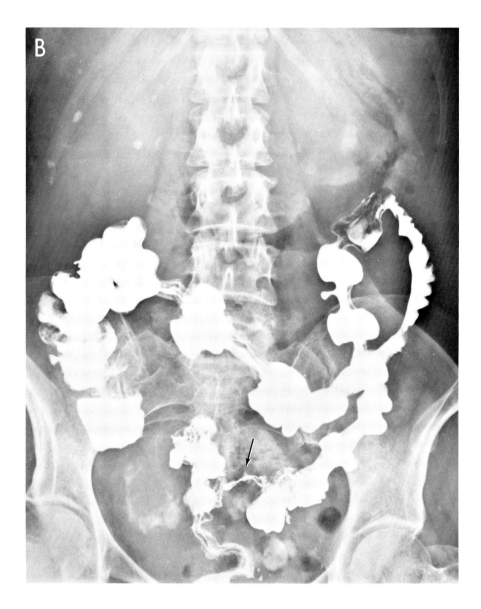

Figure 103 · Papillary Adenocarcinoma / 245

Figure 104.—Cystadenocarcinoma with metastases.

A, anteroposterior projection: Revealing large clumps of psammomatous calcification (**x**) in an ovarian neoplasm in the pelvis. Residual colon barium and bladder contrast (**y**) provide comparison of densities.

B, left posterior oblique projection: Demonstrating sigmoid colon displacement and predominantly anterior location of the tumor.

C, anteroposterior view during intravenous urography: Disclosing several calcified hepatic metastases (**arrows**).

D, posteroanterior chest study: Delineating several tiny calcified pulmonary metastases (**arrows**) and hepatic metastases superimposed on the liver in the right upper abdomen.

A painless abdominal mass was responsible for hospitalization of this patient, age 51. She had no other complaints. Surgery revealed a serous cystadenocarcinoma of the ovary with metastases. No skeletal metastases were present.

Figure 104, courtesy of Dr. C. Colangelo, Alexian Brothers Hospital, San Jose, Calif.

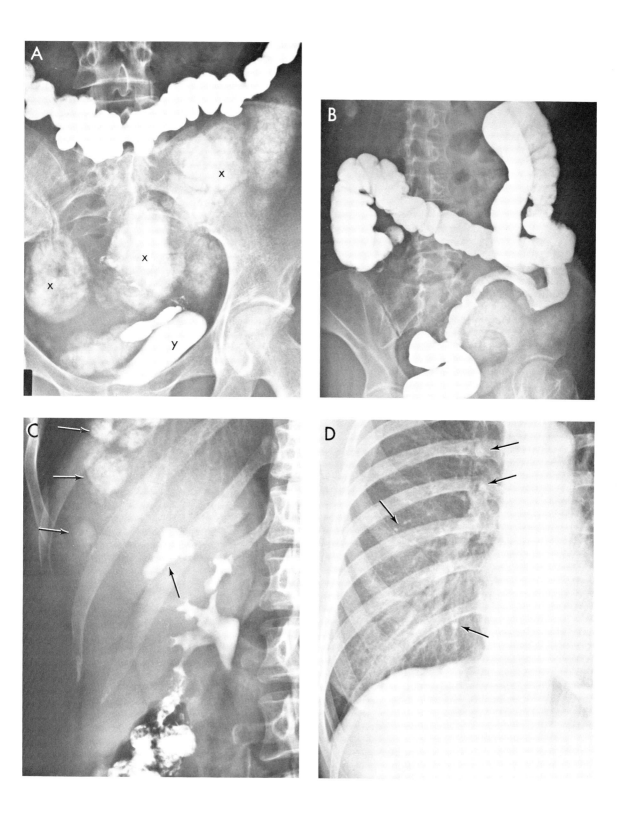

Figure 104 · Cystadenocarcinoma with Metastases / 247

Figure 105.—Bilateral papillary serous cystadenocarcinoma.

Plain film, anteroposterior projection: Revealing bilateral ovarian neoplasms of nearly uniform density due to psammomatous calcification. Though this appearance is somewhat unusual, bilateral tumors are relatively common.

At age 43, this patient had ascites that developed progressively over two to three months without accompanying symptoms. A subtotal hysterectomy had been performed 10 years previously. Radiographic examination demonstrated "bilateral calcified masses." At surgery 5 liters of yellowish ascitic fluid was obtained and bilateral 4 × 5 cm papillary serous cystadenocarcinomas of the ovaries were removed.

Figure 105, courtesy of Dr. H. Ogden, Alameda Hospital, Alameda, Calif.; previously published by Noonan, C. D.: Radiol. Clin. North America 3:375, 1965.

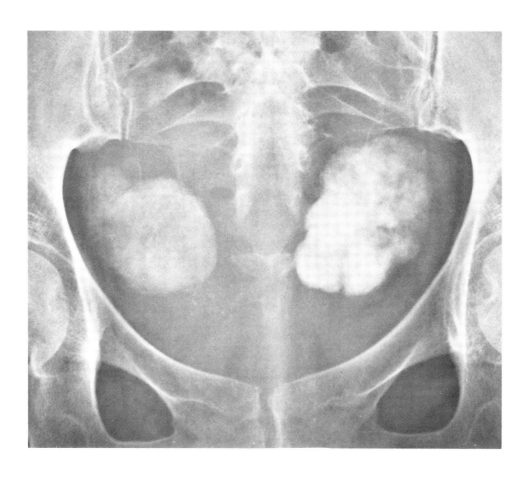

Figure 105 · Papillary Serous Cystadenocarcinoma / 249

Figure 106.—Papillary cystadenocarcinoma with metastases and calcification.

A, plain film of abdomen, anteroposterior projection: Revealing large amorphous clumps of psammomatous calcification in the papillary ovarian cystadenocarcinoma of the pelvis and abdomen. Note metastases in the right and left lobes of the liver (**arrows**). The patient had taken no barium or opaque medication previous to this study.

(*Continued* on page 252).

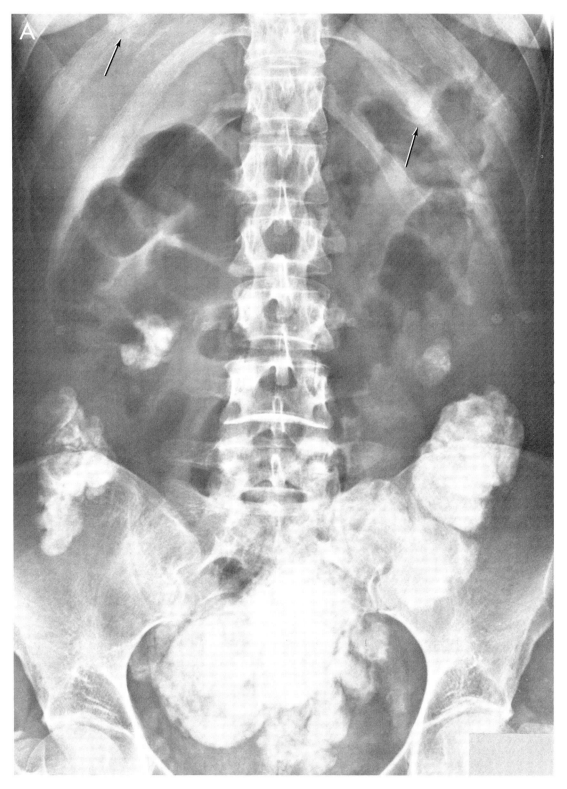

Figure 106 · Papillary Cystadenocarcinoma / 251

Figure 106 (cont.).—Papillary cystadenocarcinoma with metastases and calcification.

B, chest film: Showing psammomatous calcification (**arrow**) in a left apical pulmonary metastasis.

Diarrhea for one year and left leg swelling for four months led to pelvic laparotomy and oophorectomy in 1947 in this 50-year-old patient. A diagnosis of papillary serous cystadenocarcinoma was established. Two courses of radiation therapy followed. In 1962, because of massive tumor recurrence, frozen pelvis, nonfunctioning left kidney and partial sigmoid obstruction, palliative surgery was performed.

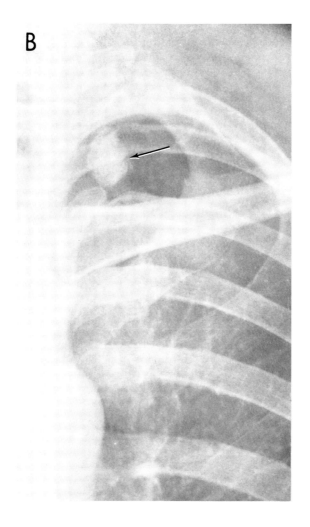

Figure 106 · Papillary Cystadenocarcinoma / 253

Figure 107.—Papillary cystadenocarcinoma with calcification and ascites.

Plain film of abdomen, anteroposterior view: Showing an amorphous mass of psammomatous calcification in a papillary ovarian cystadenocarcinoma in the central and left pelvis (**x**). At times, as in this case, the calcifications almost simulate opaque fluid. Ascitic fluid in the pelvis and abdomen is obvious.

At age 35 this patient had a malignant cystic ovarian tumor removed, followed by radiation therapy. Five years later additional tumor, identified as papillary ovarian cystadenocarcinoma, was removed. Increasing abdominal discomfort, increasing girth and early intestinal obstruction led her to seek further care. A year later, at the time this film was made, a rounded calcific density, presumably metastasis, was noted in the right lower lobe of the lung. Paracentesis and intra-aortic nitrogen mustard gave some relief, but she died about 6½ years after discovery of the tumor.

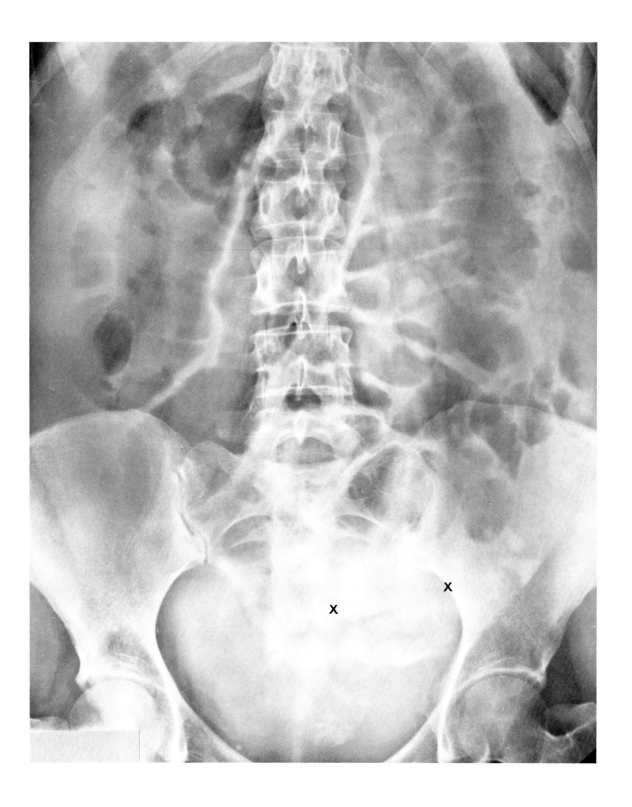

Figure 107 · Papillary Cystadenocarcinoma / 255

Figure 108.—Papillary cystadenocarcinoma with calcification.

Posteroanterior exposure after barium enema: Revealing arcuate, punctate and amorphous psammomatous calcification, at times nearly simulating a fluid of faint density, in the residual ovarian papillary cystadenocarcinoma. Note also tumor calcification in the omentum (**arrow**). Density of colon barium is striking by contrast with the faint density of the tumor calcifications (**x**).

A woman, age 55, was initially seen because of a chief complaint of abdominal enlargement. An abdominal mass was explored and found to be due to papillary ovarian cystadenocarcinoma involving both ovaries, the uterus, tubes, omentum and liver. Bilateral oophorectomy was performed. In the following three years she was hospitalized three times for bowel or biliary tract obstruction which was relieved by surgery twice and once by intubation. Nitrogen mustard was given for ascites. This film was obtained shortly before death, 3½ years after initial surgery.

Figure 108, courtesy of Drs. G. Reimer and L. R. Cooperman, Sequoia Hospital, Redwood City, Calif.

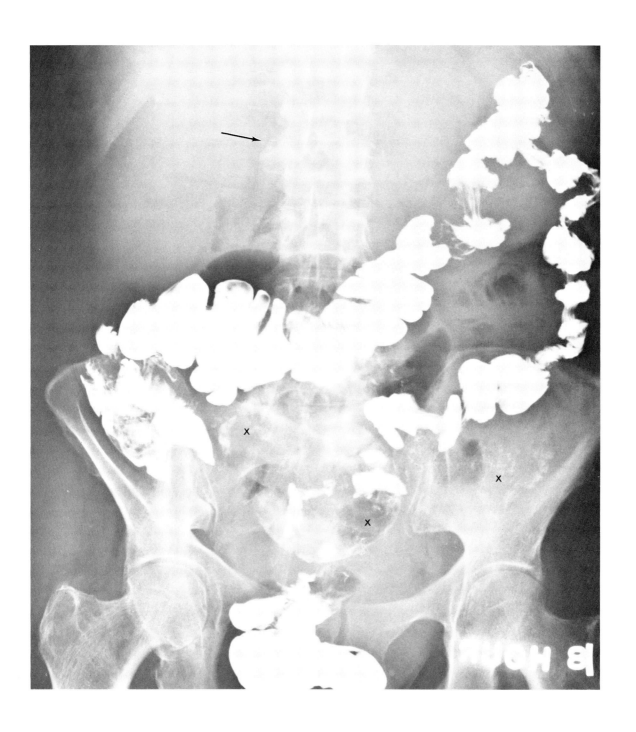

Figure 108 · Papillary Cystadenocarcinoma / 257

Figure 109.—Papillary ovarian cystadenocarcinoma spanning 20 years.

A, 2/12/47, anteroposterior exposure: Revealing whorls and clumps of calcification in an ovarian serous cystadenocarcinoma extending from the right pelvis up over the ileum.

B, 5/23/52, anteroposterior view: Showing the tumor mass and psammomatous calcification to have doubled in size in five years.

C, 1/16/59, anteroposterior view: Showing both tumor size and amount of calcification to have diminished following radiation therapy.

In 1947 this patient, age 71, was seen because of right leg swelling, believed to be due to old thrombophlebitis. Palpation revealed a firm, somewhat mobile mass in the right pelvis which on radiologic correlation at that time was thought to be a calcified fibroid or old calcified abscess. A review of earlier x-ray reports back to 1939 disclosed right pelvic calcification which had gradually increased in size. In 1951 a golf ball-size mass was removed from the left supraclavicular area and diagnosed as metastatic adenocarcinoma containing psammomatous calcification presumably from the ovary.

It was now apparent that the patient had a right ovarian carcinoma of at least 12 years' duration. Intermittent right leg swelling was managed by conservative means until 1956, when persistent swelling occurred; a 2600 rad tumor dose was given in 56 days, with disappearance of swelling and reduction of tumor size. In 1958, 2000 rads was given in 6 weeks to the pelvis and lower abdomen with excellent reduction of leg swelling. Right pleural effusion due to metastasis developed in 1959, and she died shortly thereafter at age 83.

Comment: The occasional indolent nature of this type of ovarian malignancy is well illustrated by the 20 year history in this case.

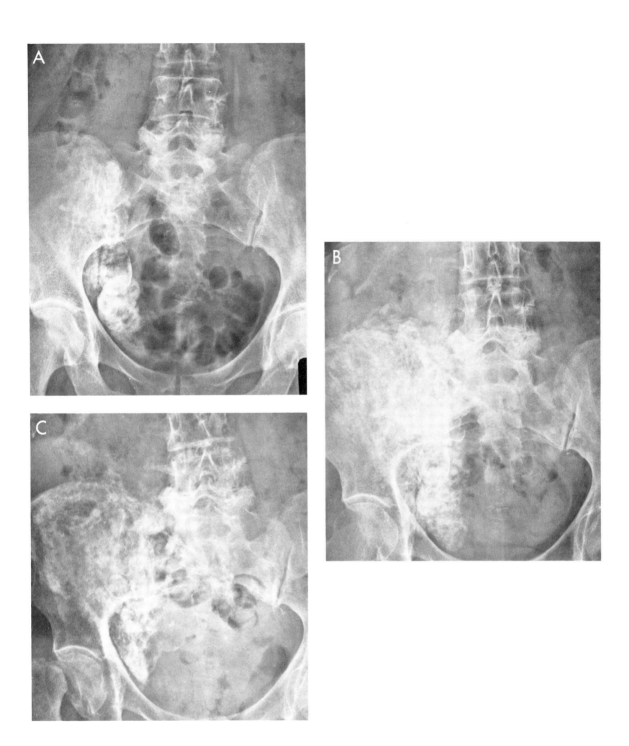

Figure 109 · Papillary Cystadenocarcinoma / 259

Figure 110.—Mucinous cystadenoma of the ovary with calcification.

A, preliminary film, anteroposterior view: Showing a thin triangular calcification and several less well identified adjacent curvilinear calcifications (**arrows**) in a pelvic mass. An artefact is seen at **x**.

B, pelvic pneumogram, posteroanterior projection: Revealing a right ovarian pelvic mass (**a**). Note calcification (**arrow**). Uterus (**b**). The left ovary is not visualized in this film.

A 42-year-old, gravida 0, para 0, obese patient was noted, on routine physical examination before going on a European tour, to have a large pelvic

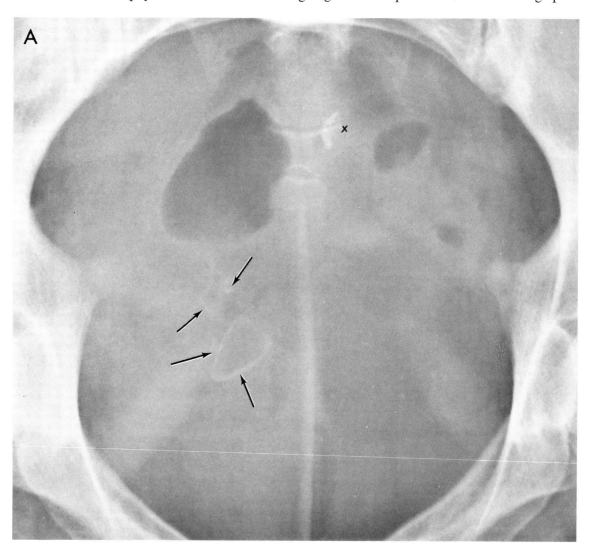

mass. Her internist thought it was a uterine fibroid, and the gynecology consultant, though uncertain, believed it was of ovarian origin. The pelvic pneumogram established the right ovary as the site of the tumor and indicated the need for surgery.

Comment: Although the literature frequently describes curvilinear calcifications in association with pseudomucinous cystadenoma and cystadenocarcinoma, most such tumors are of appendical origin, sometimes occurring after rupture (pseudomyxoma peritonei). When this tumor is of ovarian origin it very rarely calcifies. This is the only example found after a search of the files of over 15 major medical institutions and tumor registries.

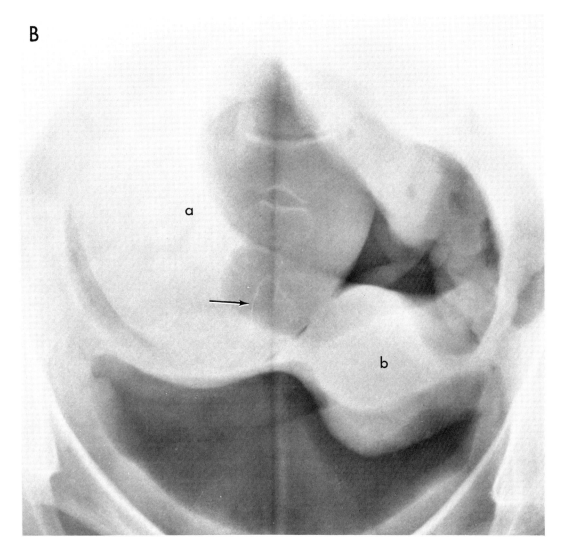

Figure 110 · Mucinous Cystadenoma: Calcification / 261

Figure 111.—Pseudomucinous cystadenocarcinoma of the ovary with osseous metaplasia.

A, preliminary film, anteroposterior view: Showing a huge pelvic and abdominal mass. Radiodensity within the tumor (**arrow**) is partially obscured by the fifth lumbar segment.

B, left posterior oblique exposure during urography: Projecting the area of osseous metaplasia free from the spine (**arrow**).

C, radiograph of surgical specimen: Demonstrating clearly the area of osseous metaplasia within the collapsed malignant cystic tumor.

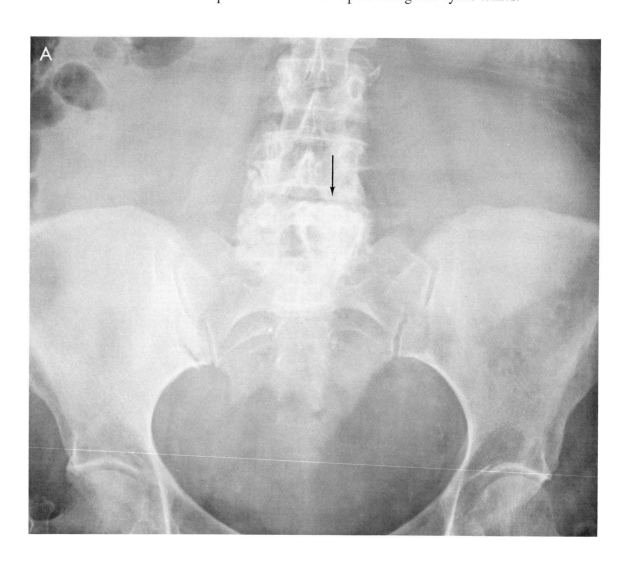

A 68-year-old, gravida 21 patient had noted scant vaginal spotting for a year or two, increasing girth and lower abdominal firmness. A very large cystic abdominal mass was palpable. The tumor extended into the left pelvic wall. Neither the origin nor any site of metastasis was revealed by preoperative work-up. A huge right ovarian mucinous cystadenocarcinoma was removed during surgery. Metastasis to various abdominal viscera and to the cervix was noted. The tumor contained localized metaplasia but no sign of a teratoma.

Comment: Areas of osseous metaplasia are not uncommonly observed microscopically but are rarely seen radiographically.

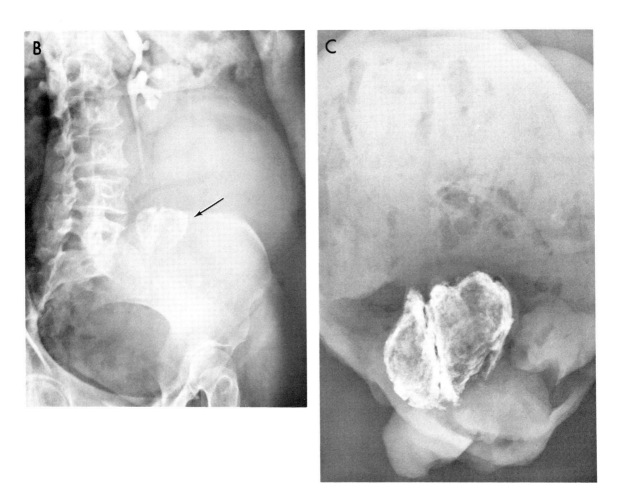

Figure 111 · Pseudomucinous Cystadenocarcinoma / 263

Figure 112.—Bilateral ovarian cystadenocarcinoma in a postmenopausal woman.

A, pelvic pneumogram, posteroanterior view; **B,** drawing of **A**: Showing marked lobular enlargement of both ovaries (**a**). Normal postmenopausal uterus (**b**); sigmoid colon (**c**). To avoid confusion between fluid-filled bowel loops and ovarian enlargement, the colon was then pneumatized (**C**).

C, pelvic pneumogram, air-inflated colon: Distinguishing the rectum and sigmoid from the bilateral ovarian neoplasms.

This gravida I, para 1 patient, age 56, experienced an uneventful menopause at age 46. Intermittent vaginal bleeding had occurred over a 15 month period. Two months before this radiographic study, dilatation and curettage had disclosed no abnormality.

The patient's large size (6 ft. 2 in., 250 lb.) limited the reliability of bimanual pelvic examination. It was believed, however, by the gynecologist that the uterus was somewhat enlarged. Pelvic pneumography was requested for clarification, and bilateral ovarian neoplasms were revealed. At surgery bilateral ovarian cystadenocarcinoma with malignant invasion of the right fallopian tube was found. The right ovary measured 10×8.5 cm; the left ovary, 14.5×9 cm. Total hysterectomy and bilateral salpingo-oophorectomy were performed, followed by radiation therapy.

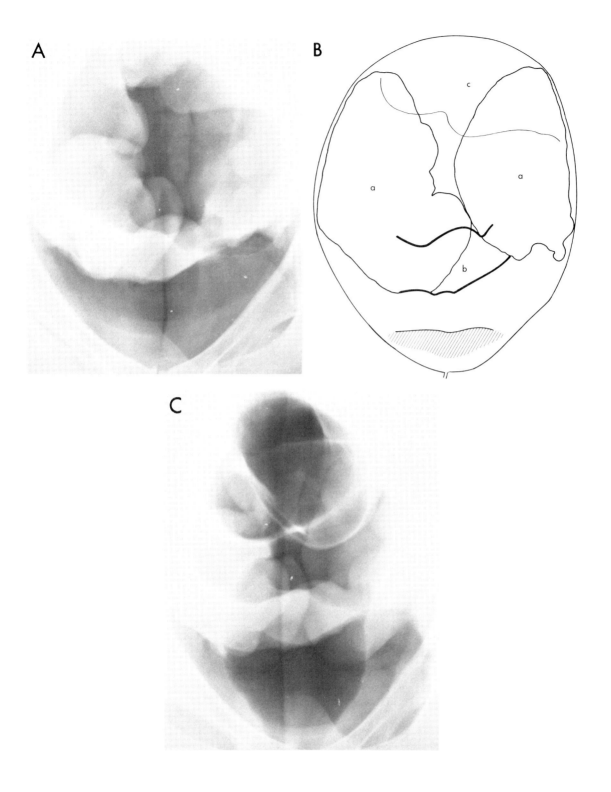

Figure 112 · Bilateral Cystadenocarcinoma / 265

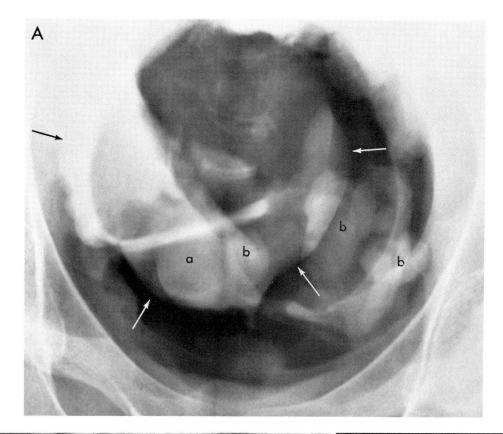

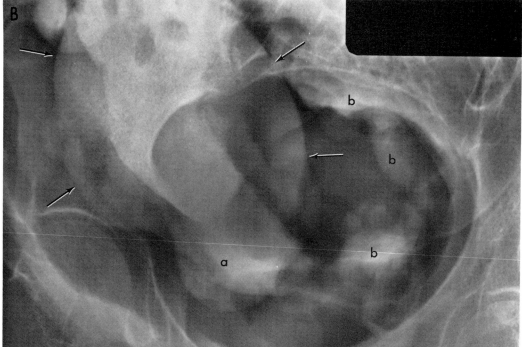

Figure 113.—Adenocarcinoma of the ovary with pelvic and abdominal metastases.

A, pelvic pneumogram, posteroanterior view: Showing a large right ovarian mass (**arrows**), with the uterus (**a**) drawn to the right and attached to the mass, and numerous pelvic tumor implants (**b**).

B, pelvic pneumogram, right anterior oblique projection: Delineating the right ovarian mass (**arrows**), the uterus attached to the mass (**a**), and implants (**b**).

C, pneumoperitoneum, left lateral decubitus projection: Revealing numerous tumor implants (**b**), a large plaque of tumor in the right upper quadrant adjacent to the right lobe of the liver and ascitic fluid-air level.

A 46-year-old woman had a history of intermittent right upper quadrant abdominal pain for four months, ascites for two months, anorexia and occasional vomiting. A firm rectal shelf was palpable and was initially believed to be secondary to a mediastinal tumor. Paracentesis yielded 6500 cc of ascitic fluid and the cytologic diagnosis of adenocarcinoma. Pelvic and abdominal pneumography identified a large right ovarian tumor and numerous pelvic and upper abdominal metastases, indicating the futility of resection. The mediastinal "tumor" was later proved to be produced by a diaphragmatic hernia. Intraperitoneal [198]Au therapy was given.

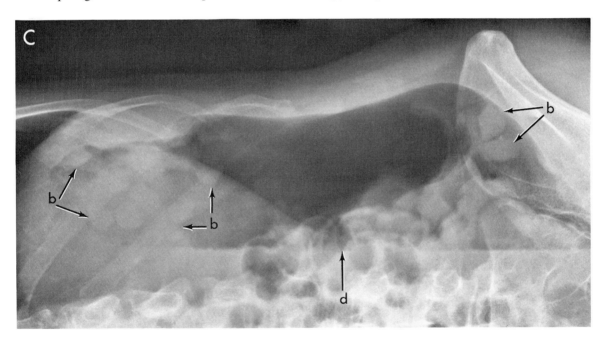

Figure 113 · **Adenocarcinoma & Metastases** / **267**

Figure 114.—Serous cystadenocarcinoma with Meigs's syndrome.

A, chest film, posteroanterior view: Showing right pleural effusion, confirmed by a right lateral decubitus exposure.

B, pelvic pneumogram, posteroanterior view: Revealing a large right ovarian mass (**a**) that falls cephalad in the 45° head-down position. Note the stretched right fallopian tube (**b**). Uterus (**c**); left ovary (**d**); left round ligament (**e**).

C, pelvic pneumogram, lateral projection: Showing the large right ovarian mass (**a**) in a pool of ascitic fluid (**arrow**). Uterus (**c**); left ovary (**d**). Ascites had not been suspected clinically.

The patient, 45, reported increasing girth, a lower abdominal mass palpable when she was supine, and a paroxysmal cough of two weeks' duration. Menses were normal, and a pregnancy test gave a negative result. Dullness in the base of the right lung was noted on physical examination, and uterine fibroids were suspected on pelvic examination. Pelvic pneumography was requested to confirm the latter. Fluid was encountered, and cytologic examination confirmed the ovarian carcinoma suspected from the radiographic evidence. The chest radiograph confirmed the presence of right pleural effusion, proved to be cytologically negative on thoracentesis. No tumor implants on the pelvic or abdominal peritoneal surfaces were seen on pneumoperitoneography or at surgery. The right ovarian tumor was $9 \times 10 \times 11$ cm and was believed to contain both serous cystadenocarcinoma and hypernephroid carcinoma with vascular invasion. Seven years after hysterectomy, bilateral oophorectomy and [198]Au therapy she was well, without recurrence.

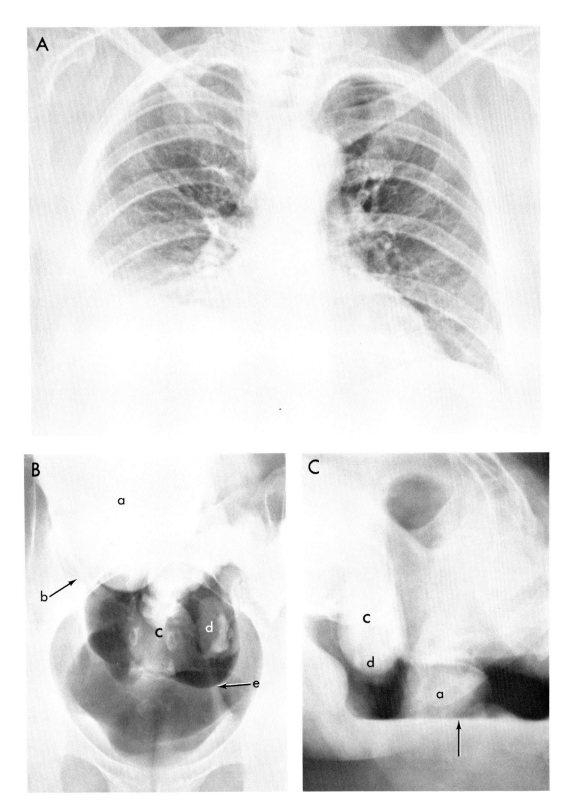

Figure 114 · Cystadenocarcinoma & Meigs's Syndrome / 269

Figure 115.—Ovarian carcinomatosis.

A, pelvic pneumogram, with central beam perpendicular to the floor, posteroanterior projection; **B,** drawing of **A:** Showing the uterus (**a**) eccentrically positioned to the left of the midline. Multiple metastases are obvious in rectouterine and vesicouterine pouches as well as on the broad ligament and uterus (**stippled areas**). Bladder (**b**). There is residual barium in the colon.

A 71-year-old woman was seen because of her concern that a malignancy might explain her moderate weight loss. She was reassured after careful examination. Two months later she returned because of continued weight loss, anorexia and protuberant abdomen. No positive physical abnormalities were detected. A gastrointestinal series, barium enema and small bowel series were uninformative. Ascites was encountered during peritoneal inflation for pelvic pneumography. Pelvic carcinomatosis was diagnosed radiographically and confirmed as adenocarcinoma on cytologic examination. The patient died within two months.

Comment: Although this is believed to be due to an ovarian primary, it is possible that it represents metastatic adenocarcinoma from elsewhere. In any event, the advanced state of the disease and the futility of surgery are obvious.

A

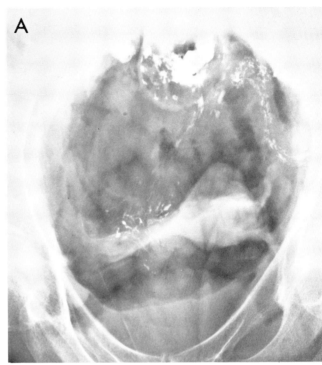

B

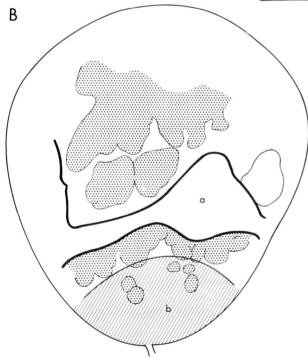

Figure 115 · Ovarian Carcinomatosis / 271

Figure 116.—Bilateral ovarian papillary adenocarcinoma with peritoneal implants.

A, pelvic pneumogram, posteroanterior view; **B,** drawing of **A**: Delineating bilateral ovarian carcinoma (**a**), normal uterus (**b**) and sigmoid colon (**c**). There are nodular metastases (**stippled areas**) on the uterine isthmus and sigmoid colon.

C, pelvic pneumogram, left anterior oblique projection: **D,** drawing of **C**: Demonstrating the metastases on the sigmoid to better advantage.

A recent history of conspicuous epigastric fullness and discomfort in the right upper quadrant marked the onset of symptoms in this patient of 43. Even a small quantity of food or fluid caused bloating and epigastric pressure. Nausea and anorexia followed. Physical, including pelvic, examination gave essentially negative results. Three days later ascites was clinically evident and pelvic pneumography was ordered. Cytologic examination of ascitic fluid obtained during pelvic pneumography confirmed the radiologic diagnosis of ovarian carcinomatosis (papillary adenocarcinoma). Radioactive colloidal [198]Au and external ^{60}Co therapy was given. Bilateral oophorectomy and supracervical hysterectomy were done. Two weeks later gastroenterostomy and cholecystoduodenostomy were required to bypass a duodenal obstruction by the tumor. She died eight months after discovery of the tumor.

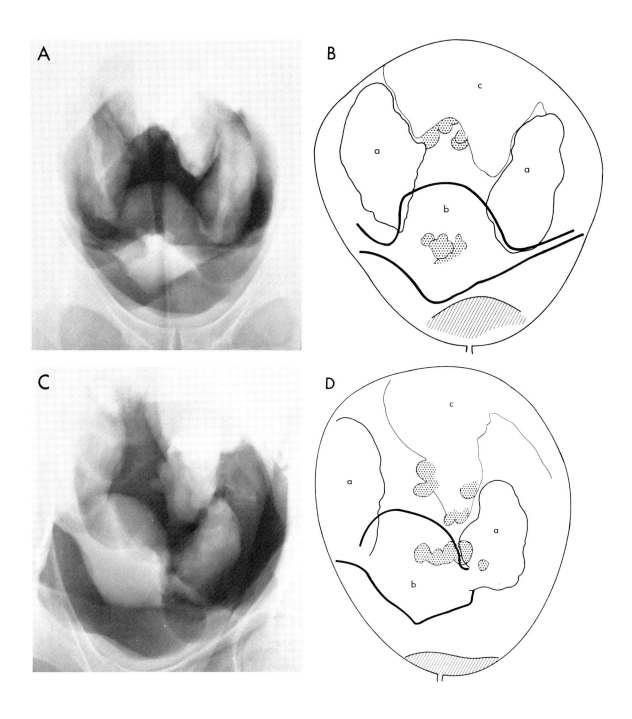

Figure 116 · Bilateral Papillary Adenocarcinoma / 273

Figure 117.—Bilateral mesonephroma: pelvic pneumograms.

A, posteroanterior projection: Showing a moderately large right ovarian mass (**a**), marked lobular enlargement of the left ovary (**b**) and normal uterus (**c**).

B, right anterior oblique projection: Delineating the posterior lateral outline of the right ovarian tumor (**a**). The entirety of the left ovarian tumor (**b**) is not seen, but the ovarian origin is clear. Uterus (**c**).

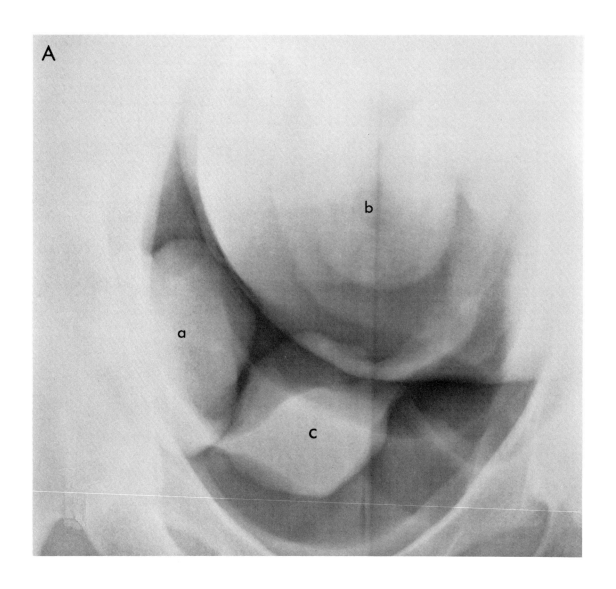

This gravida 0 patient of 44 had normal menstruation except for slight dysmenorrhea the first day. On physical examination the distinction between uterine fibroids and ovarian tumor could not be made. Following pelvic pneumography, surgery was performed and a 7 cm right and 12 cm left ovarian mesonephroma removed. No capsular breakthrough or metastasis was seen.

Comment: By resolving the question of ovarian vs. uterine origin of the pelvic mass and demonstrating the clearcut presence of bilateral ovarian tumors, the need for laparotomy was established.

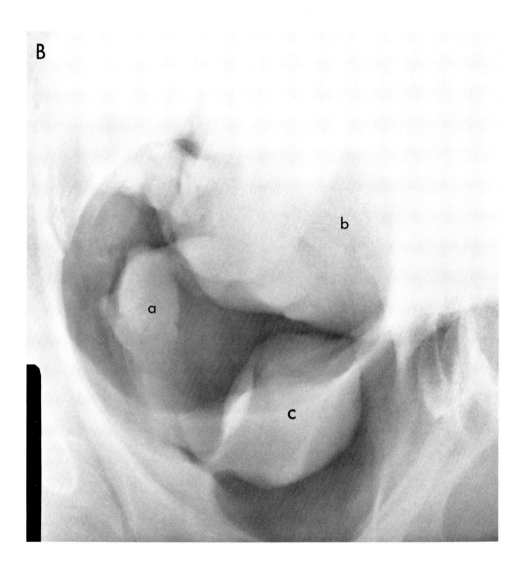

Figure 117 · Bilateral Mesonephroma / 275

Figure 118.—Recurrent papillary adenocarcinoma of the ovary following surgery and radiation therapy.

Pelvic pneumogram, posteroanterior projection: Showing numerous tumor masses (**a**) and metastatic implants (**b**) in the rectouterine pouch and uterine operative site.

At age 46 this woman had a total hysterectomy and bilateral salpingo-oophorectomy for poorly differentiated ovarian papillary adenocarcinoma with several pelvic implants. She subsequently received a 6000 rad radiation dose to the pelvis and lower abdomen in 63 days. Two years later, tumor recurrence in the pelvis was suspected, but differentiation from radiation effect was difficult. After recurrent tumor was demonstrated on the pelvic pneumogram she received systemic chemotherapy.

Comment: Gas inflation of the rectum and sigmoid colon and subsequent repeat prone and horizontal beam lateral films of the pelvis are helpful in distinguishing between fluid-filled bowel and tumor if there is any doubt.

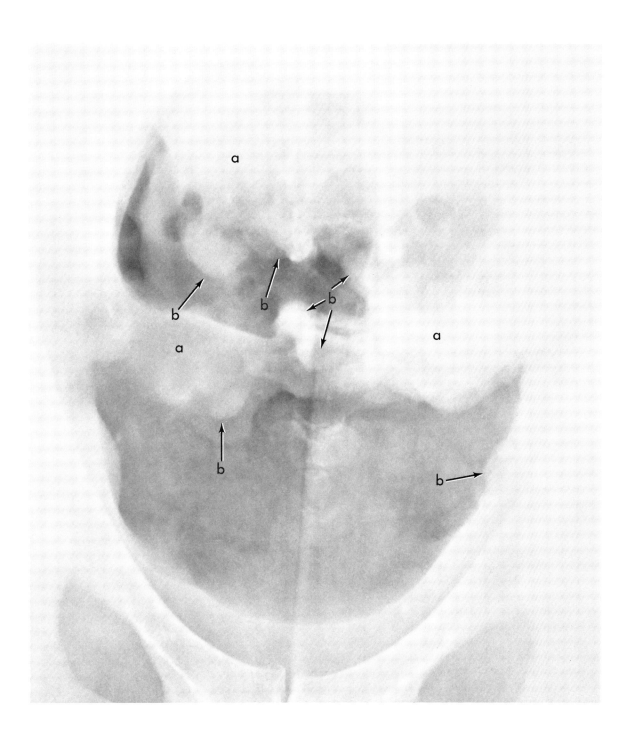

Figure 118 · Recurrent Papillary Adenocarcinoma / 277

Figure 119.—Reticulum cell sarcoma of the ovary.

Pelvic pneumogram, posteroanterior projection: Showing evidence of previous hysterectomy, a large right ovarian mass (**a**) and the left ovary (**b**) moderately enlarged. Residual barium is seen in the bowel. Urinary bladder (**c**).

This 46-year-old woman was hospitalized because of bladder fullness and urinary frequency. Anemia and a central pelvic mass were the most significant findings. There was a history of vaginal hysterectomy. During laparotomy the large right ovarian mass was identified as reticulum cell sarcoma, and she was given 4500 rads to the pelvis and a dose of 2200 rads to the paraortic region. A year later a similar tumor was found in the liver and nitrogen mustard and transfusions were given. She died of widespread metastases 15 months after the initial laparotomy.

Comment: Whether this tumor was primary in the ovaries or metastatic is moot. The fact is that metastatic neoplasms of the ovary are moderately common and may come from any source, the most common being tumors of the reproductive and gastrointestinal tracts. None have pathognomonic radiographic features.

Figure 119, courtesy of Dr. J. J. McCort, Valley Medical Center, San Jose, Calif.

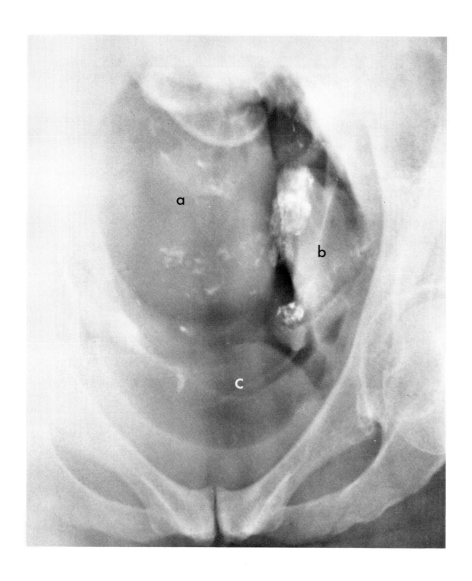

Figure 119 · Reticulum Cell Sarcoma / 279

Figure 120.—Papillary cystadenocarcinoma of the ovary in a child.

A, anteroposterior abdominal study: Revealing a huge smooth-bordered abdominal mass.

B, anteroposterior exposure after barium: Demonstrating that the tumor is extrinsic to the digestive and urinary tracts.

For one month this girl of 6 years had had abdominal swelling and mild constipation. A large cystic mass was palpable. Extrinsic displacement of the gastrointestinal tract was seen on gastrointestinal and barium enema examinations. The chest and urinary tract were normal radiographically, and blood and urine examinations showed no abnormalities. At operation the tumor was found to originate in the right ovary and to be confined to this organ. A right salpingo-oophorectomy was performed. The pathologist's diagnosis was papillary cystadenocarcinoma of the ovary.

Comment: Ovarian cysts and neoplasms are not rare in infants and children.

Figure 120, courtesy of Dr. J. J. McCort, Valley Medical Center, San Jose, Calif.

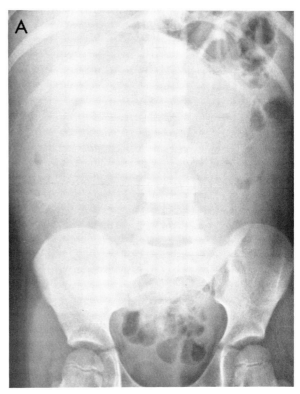

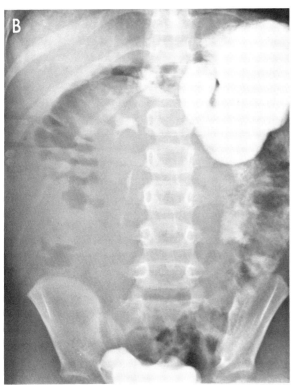

Figure 120 · Cystadenocarcinoma in a Child / 281

Figure 121.—Bilateral ovarian adenocarcinoma: pelvic angiograms.

A, early arterial phase, with catheter tip above aortic bifurcation, anteroposterior projection: Delineating the uterine arteries (**4**) with hypertrophic and tortuous intramural tributaries, uterine isthmus (**a**) and early filling of right adnexal tumor vessels (**b**).

B, late arterial phase: Revealing tumor vessels in the right ovarian tumor (**c**). Uterine isthmus (**a**). The left ovarian tumor is not confidently seen.

(*Continued* on page 284).

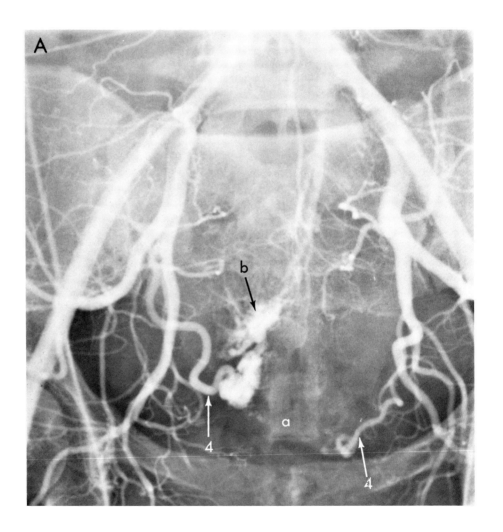

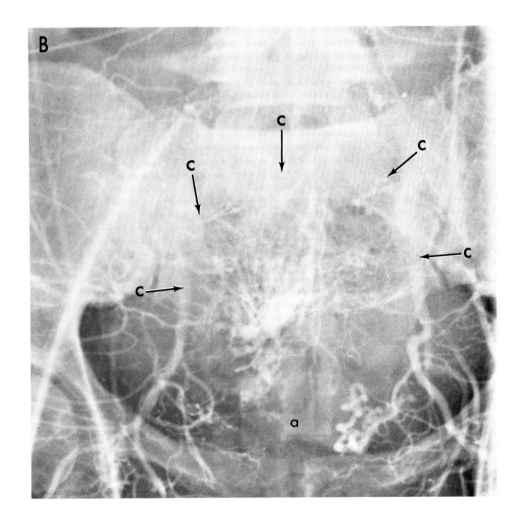

Figure 121 · Bilateral Adenocarcinoma / 283

Figure 121 (cont.).—Bilateral ovarian adenocarcinoma: pelvic angiograms.

C, a second injection with catheter tip at the level of the third lumbar segment, slight left posterior oblique projection: Demonstrating enlarged right uterine artery with tortuous intramural portion (**4**). Enlarged right and left ovarian arteries (**10**) are now seen which correlate with the bilateral ovarian neoplasms found.

A 31-year-old patient had a six month history of irregular vaginal bleeding and dysmenorrhea and increasing girth. Uterine fibroids had been suspected three months previously. Now a large, firm right adnexal mass and a softer left adnexal mass were palpable. Ovarian vs. uterine origin of the masses? Bilateral ovarian and appendical adenocarcinoma was found at surgery.

Comment: The difficulty of distinguishing between benign and malignant neoplasms and at times whether the mass arises in the ovary, uterus or adnexa often seriously limits the practical usefulness of angiography. Considerable difference in enthusiasm for this procedure exists among radiologists.

Figure 121, courtesy of Drs. C. Rådberg and I. Wickbom, Gothenberg, Sweden.

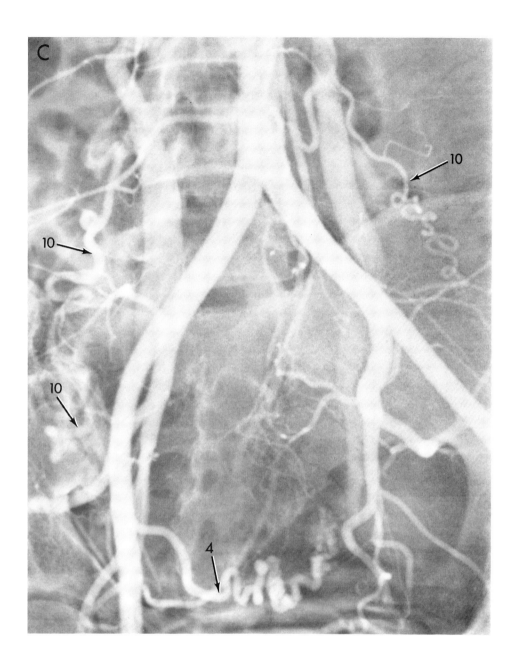

Figure 121 · **Bilateral Adenocarcinoma** / **285**

Figure 122.—Dysgerminoma: pelvic angiograms.

A, midarterial phase, anteroposterior projection: Revealing a large right adnexal mass, uterine arteries (**4**), ovarian artery (**10**) and a large plexus of tumor vessels in the right adnexal area arising from the uterine and right ovarian arteries.

(*Continued* on page 288).

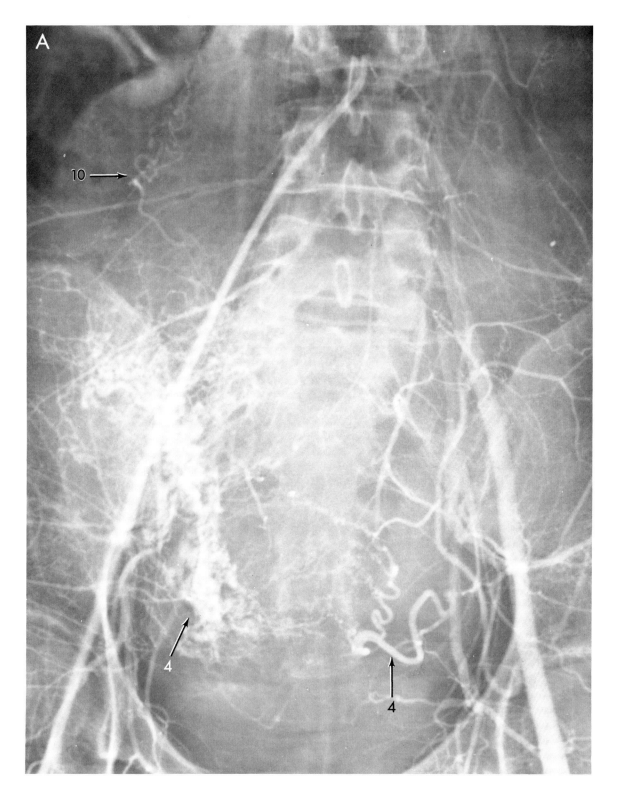

Figure 122 · Ovarian Dysgerminoma / 287

Figure 122 (cont.).—Dysgerminoma: pelvic angiograms.

B, late arterial phase: With the intramural arcades delineating the central uterine position (**a**). An enormous right ovarian dysgerminoma is outlined by tumor vessels (**arrows**).

The patient, 25, had abdominal pain, recent irregular vaginal bleeding and had noted a mass in the right abdomen for over a year. The mass, clinically mobile and well delineated, was believed to be an ovarian cystic tumor.

Figure 122, courtesy of Drs. C. Rådberg and I. Wickbom, Gothenberg, Sweden.

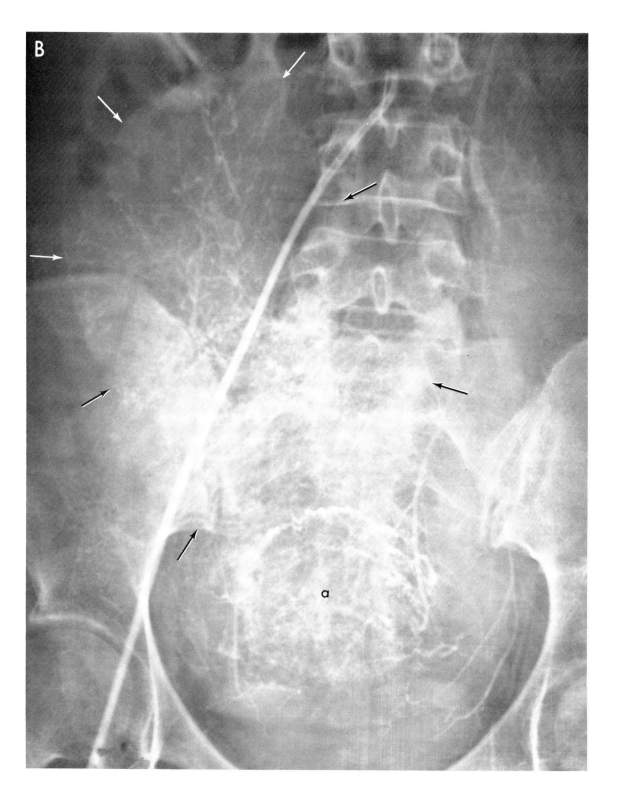

Figure 122 · Ovarian Dysgerminoma / 289

Figure 123.—Pseudotumors of the pelvis due to fluid-filled small bowel loops associated with regional enteritis.

Postevacuation barium enema study, posteroanterior view: Delineating two rounded masses (**arrows**) in the pelvis.

A woman of 74 had severe abdominal cramps for 24 hours and was unable to defecate. Similar episodes had occurred infrequently during the previous 10 months. Sigmoidoscopy was not revealing. Two cystlike lesions were identified in the pelvis on the flat abdominal plate and an ovarian cyst was suspected on clinical examination. Barium enema disclosed an area of terminal ileal narrowing. At surgery, adherent distended small bowel loops were found in the pelvis which accounted for the two masses seen in the radiograph. A short segment of regional enteritis involved the terminal ileum. The ovaries were small and contained no cysts.

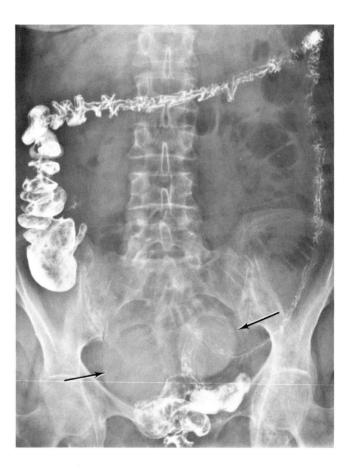

Figure 124.—Left ovarian pseudotumor due to fluid-filled sigmoid loop: pelvic pneumograms.

A, posteroanterior projection: Revealing a lobular homogeneous density in the posterior left pelvis (**a**). Ovarian enlargement vs. fluid-filled bowel? Uterus (**b**); right ovary (**c**).

B, after pneumatization of rectum and sigmoid, posteroanterior exposure: Dispelling the suspicion of left ovarian enlargement and proving that the density is produced by a fluid-filled sigmoid loop. The poorly defined left ovary (**d**) is now uncovered by gas-filled bowel.

This gravida II, para 2 patient, age 28, had had left lower quadrant crampy pain for two or three weeks. Pain seemed to intensify as the day progressed. She had no nausea or vomiting. A left adnexal mass believed to be a cyst was felt by two different examiners. The fluid-filled sigmoid colon demonstrated on the pelvic pneumogram probably accounted for the clinical illusion of an adnexal mass. Inflation of the rectum and sigmoid established that this was not due to ovarian or tubal enlargement. The pelvic pain subsequently disappeared.

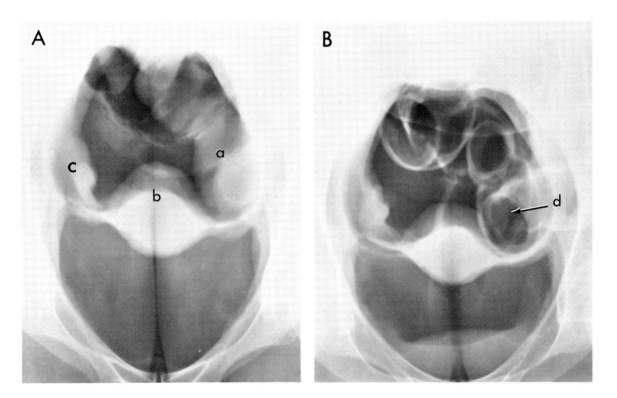

Figure 124 · Pseudotumor: Sigmoid Loop / 291

Figure 125.—Pseudotumor of the left ovary produced by fluid-filled sigmoid loop: pelvic pneumograms.

A, posteroanterior projection: Showing the right ovary (**a**) to be about four times normal size. There appears to be left ovarian enlargement (**b**). Uterus (**c**).

B, left anterior oblique projection: Confirming presence of the right ovarian mass (**a**). The left ovarian mass (**b**) seen in **A** contains intraluminal gas identifying it as bowel. The left ovary (**d**) is now clearly seen.

C, lateral view, with horizontal beam: Showing the fluid-filled sigmoid loop (**arrows**) which in **A** simulates left ovarian enlargement. Uterus (**c**).

The presence of right lower quadrant pain and the clinical suspicion of a cul-de-sac mass by the gynecologist prompted pelvic pneumography in this patient of 42 years. Bilateral ovarian masses were diagnosed on the pelvic pneumogram, though in retrospect air inflation of the rectum and sigmoid should have been carried out. Surgery two weeks after pneumography demonstrated a fluid-filled sigmoid loop secondary to intestinal adhesions in the left posterior pelvis. The left ovary was buried in small adhesions and attached to the sigmoid colon. The right ovary was only slightly enlarged (4 × 5 cm) and contained some small cysts. Apparently the right ovarian cyst had leaked its contents and diminished greatly in size in the interval prior to surgery.

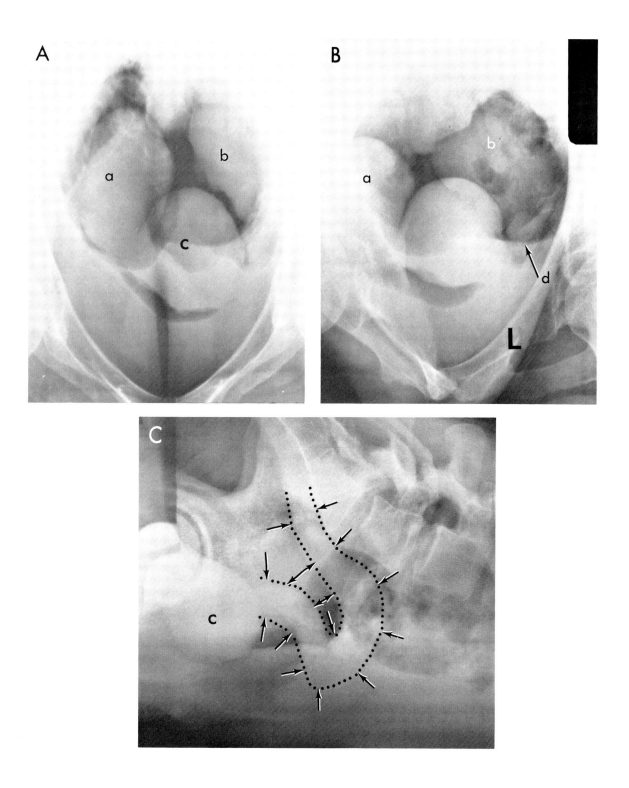

Figure 125 · Pseudotumor: Sigmoid Loop / 293

Figure 126.—Hydrosalpinx with tubal-ovarian mass.

A, pelvic pneumogram, posteroanterior projection; and **B,** drawing of **A:** Showing a left tubal-ovarian mass (hydrosalpinx) (**a**) and cystic left ovary (**b**) distinctly separated from, but adherent to, the sigmoid colon (**c**). The uterus is large for a postmenopausal patient and is positioned eccentrically to the right (**d**). Small postmenopausal right ovary (**e**); fallopian tube (**f**).

This postmenopausal patient, age 53, had an established long-term history of diverticulitis. While taking estrogens for postmenopausal symptoms she was hospitalized with a one year history of vaginal spotting. A slightly tender 6–8 cm mass was suspected in the left adnexa, but the findings were equivocal. The presence of diverticulitis raised the question of sigmoid vs. reproductive tract abnormality. Pelvic pneumography was performed to clarify this question.

Dilatation and curettage provided evidence of a very well differentiated adenocarcinoma of the endometrium with superficial invasion and marked adenomyosis. The tubal-ovarian origin of the left adnexal mass was verified at surgery, when a tortuous left hydrosalpinx and left ovarian cyst were found. Adhesions extended between the sigmoid and the left ovary, presumably the result of the old diverticulitis.

Comment: The difficulty in distinguishing between alimentary tract and reproductive tract disease is common on pelvic examination. Pelvic pneumography is often useful in clarifying the site or origin of disease. The enlarged uterus in this case was predominantly due to adenomyosis. In cases such as this a combined pelvic pneumogram and uterosalpingogram may be helpful in determining tubal involvement.

A

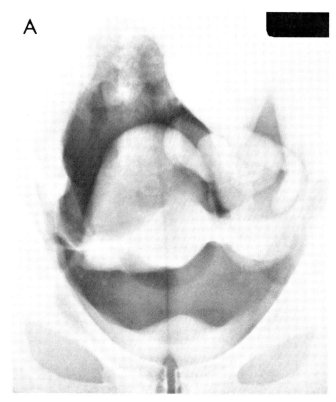

B

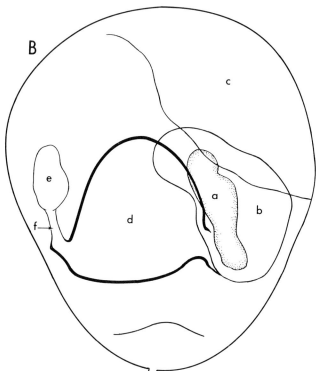

Figure 126 · Pseudotumor: Hydrosalpinx / 295

Figure 127.—Sigmoid diverticulitis producing pseudotumor.

A, pelvic pneumogram, posteroanterior projection: Delineating a mass (**a**) in the posterior left pelvis separate from the uterus (**b**) and atrophic left ovary (**c**).

B, pelvic pneumogram, lateral view: Showing the mass (**a**) posterior to and separate from the uterus (**b**). Some extraperitoneal N_2O is seen (**d**).

C, left posterior oblique view after barium enema: Revealing extensive diverticulosis.

D, lateral projection after barium enema: Demonstrating sigmoid diverticulosis. Compare with the lateral view in **B.**

A 69-year-old woman with a history of diverticulosis complained of pelvic pressure on straining and some accompanying urinary frequency and stress incontinence. An irregular, poorly defined, slightly tender mass was palpable in the posterior cul-de-sac. Pelvic pneumography and barium enema confirmed the clinical suspicion that this was a pseudotumor produced by diverticulitis.

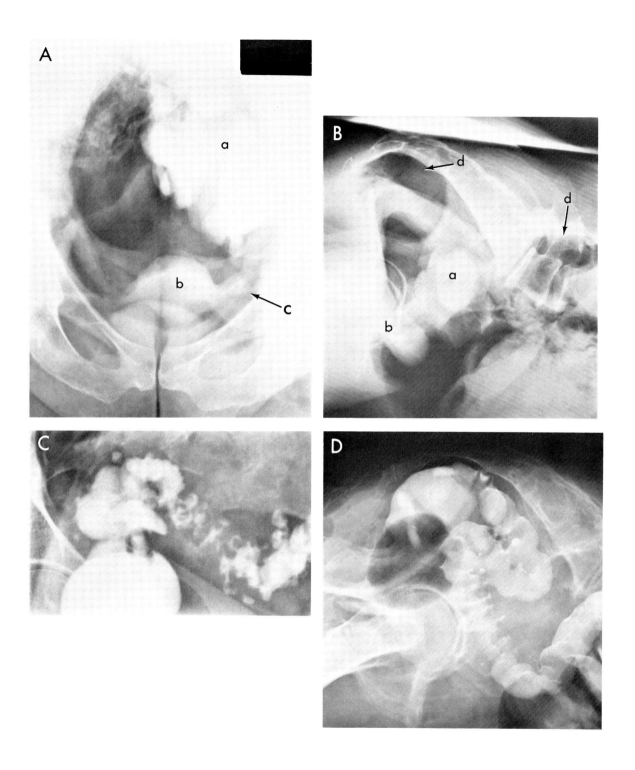

Figure 127 · Pseudotumor: Diverticulitis / 297

Figure 128.—Ectopic, tubal pregnancy producing ovarian pseudotumor.

Pelvic pneumogram, posteroanterior projection: Showing an oval mass (**a**) adjacent to the left ovary (**b**). Left fallopian tube (**c**).

Ectopic pregnancy was suspected in this 23-year-old patient. Four months previously, a right tubal pregnancy had occurred and right salpingectomy followed. Tenderness in the left adnexa and rectouterine pouch was noted, but no mass was palpable. After radiographic confirmation of a tubal mass, surgery was performed and the diagnosis of ectopic, tubal pregnancy confirmed.

Comment: A palpable mass is present in only one-third to one-half of patients with ectopic pregnancy. Since the clinical diagnosis is often difficult, radiographic confirmation of the mass becomes most helpful.

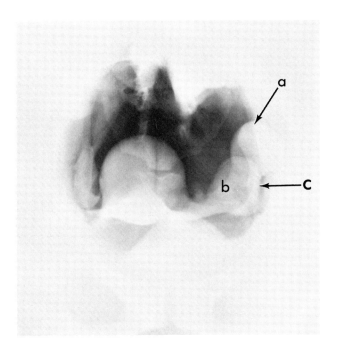

Figure 129.—Ectopic kidney producing a pelvic mass.

A, pelvic pneumogram during excretory urography, posteroanterior view; **B,** drawing of **A:** Depicting the pelvic kidney (**a**), enlarged uterus (**b**), slightly enlarged left ovary (**c**) and tiny right ovary (**d**).

In a 33-year-old woman, a mass was discovered on pelvic examination. An excretory urogram showed an ectopic pelvic position of the left kidney. To make sure that the pelvic kidney explained the palpable mass, a pelvic pneumogram was obtained. The uterus was twice normal size but clearly separated from the pelvic kidney.

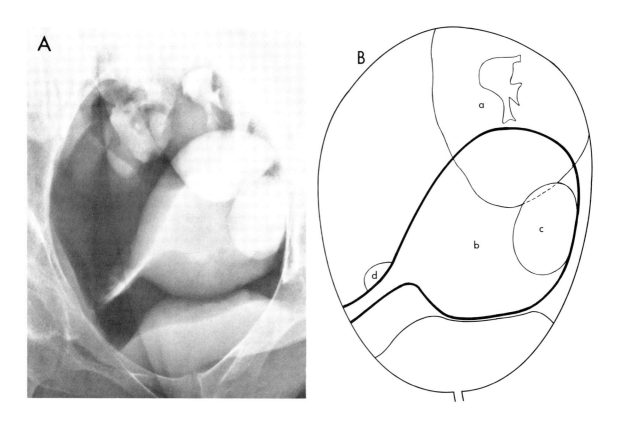

Figure 129 · Pseudotumor: Ectopic Kidney / 299

Figure 130.—Endometriosis.

A, pelvic pneumogram, posteroanterior projection; **B,** drawing of **A:** Revealing a conglomerate mass involving the uterus (**a**), ovaries (**b**) and sigmoid colon (**c**) and filling the posterior pelvis. Such a conglomerate mass is typical of endometriosis. Note cystic enlargement of the right ovary.

A gravida IV, para 4 patient, age 41, was asymptomatic except for "irritation" on voiding and slight increase in urinary frequency. Menstruation was normal. A urologist noted a mass the size of a lemon in the right side of the pelvis; this was verified by a gynecologist, who thought a cyst was present and attached to the uterus. Demonstration on the pelvic pneumogram of the conglomerate mass led to diagnosis of endometriosis, confirmed at surgery. The right ovarian enlargement was due to a corpus luteum cyst, but extensive changes of endometriosis were present. Hysterectomy and bilateral salpingo-oophorectomy were performed.

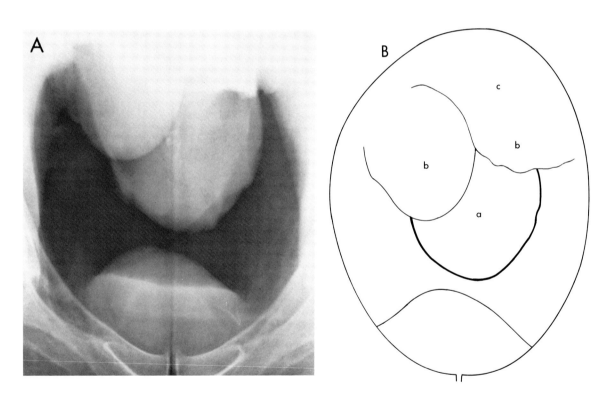

Figure 131.—Endometrioma.

A, pelvic pneumogram, posteroanterior projection; **B,** drawing of **A:** Delineating a large right ovarian mass (**a**), slightly enlarged, cystic left ovary (**b**), uterus (**c**) and sigmoid colon (**d**).

A gravida I, para 1 woman, age 28, had had right pelvic pain for two months. Menses were regular and she was normal otherwise. A 6 × 7 cm right adnexal mass was palpable on bimanual pelvic examination and pelvic pneumography was ordered. Twelve days later, surgery revealed a large endometrioma of the right ovary filling the cul-de-sac of Douglas and adhering to the right pelvic wall and posterior aspect of the right broad ligament. The left ovary contained several small follicular cysts. The uterus was normal.

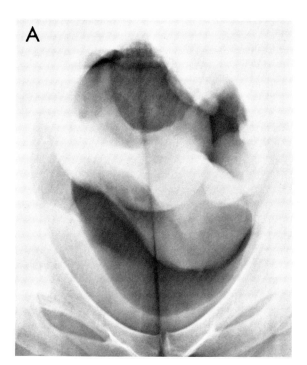
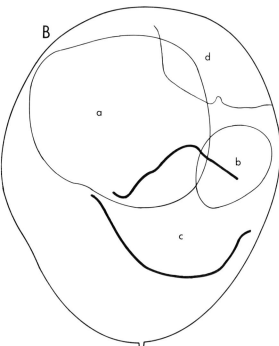

Figure 131 · Endometrioma / 301

Figure 132.—Endometrioma.

A, pelvic pneumogram, posteroanterior projection; **B,** drawing of **A:** Showing a large, lobular right ovarian endometrioma (**a**); a moderate-size endometrioma attached to the left ovary (**b**); normal uterus displaced to the left pelvis (**c**); urinary bladder (**d**); sigmoid colon (**e**).

At age 37 this woman had mild right lower abdominal pain. The uterus was thought to be two or three times normal size on pelvic examination. After pelvic pneumography demonstrated bilateral ovarian enlargement, surgery disclosed bilateral endometriomas. That on the right was 9×10 cm in diameter; the left one, which was attached to the ovary, measured 4×5 cm. Right salpingo-oophorectomy and left ovarian cystectomy were performed.

Comment: These masses are unusually large for endometriomas and lack the surrounding adhesions which usually accompany this "tumor."

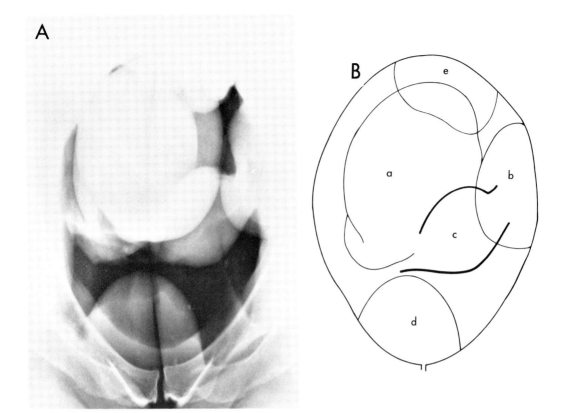

Figure 132 · Endometriomas / 303

Figure 133.—Endometrioma of the left ovary.

A, pelvic pneumogram, posteroanterior projection: Demonstrating a conglomerate mass in the central and posterior portions of the pelvis comprised of uterus, enlarged ovaries and sigmoid colon. The right round ligament (**a**) extends to the uterus (**b**).

B, pelvic pneumogram, left anterior oblique view: Showing the uterine-ovarian portion of the mass (**c**) attached to the partially gas-filled rectum and sigmoid (**d**).

C, after barium enema, left posterior oblique view: Revealing luminal narrowing of the lower sigmoid colon (**arrows**) produced by encircling endometriosis.

D, after barium enema, lateral view: Showing constancy of the sigmoid narrowing (**arrows**).

A para 2 patient, age 41, had had abdominal tenderness and pain coincident with menstruation during the previous three cycles. A tender 5–6 cm mass was palpable above the left vaginal fornix. At surgery a 6×7.5 cm endometrioma of the left ovary was found, with adhesions between the sigmoid colon and the endometrioma. The left ovary was buried in the posterior aspect of the left broad ligament. The right ovary was normal but contained several cysts. Endometriosis also involved the anterior aspect of the uterus and the bowel.

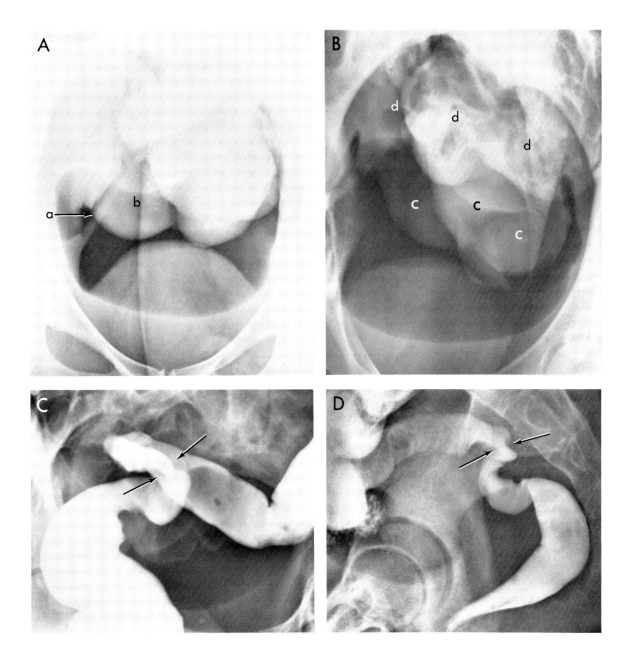

Figure 133 · Endometrioma / 305

Figure 134.—Endometrioma of the left ovary with adhesions and right fallopian tube anomaly.

A, pelvic pneumogram, posteroanterior projection: **B,** drawing of **A:** Demonstrating a large left ovarian mass (**a**) and the uterine fundus (**b**) retracted to the left by adhesions (**arrows**) which attach it to the lateral pelvic wall and the left ovarian mass. The fusiform mass (**c**) proved to be a fibroma of the round ligament. The right ovary is slightly enlarged (**d**).

C, combined uterosalpingogram and pelvic pneumogram: Delineating the patent left fallopian tube (**arrow**) and nonfilling of the right tube.

Gross menstrual irregularity and menorrhagia prompted this 23-year-old patient to seek medical care. She had also been infertile during two marriages which lasted a total of three years. The uterus and right ovary were believed to be normal on pelvic examination, but a 6 cm mass was palpable in the region of the left ovary. Endometrioma of the left ovary, uterine adhesions and failure of filling of the right tube were diagnosed on radiographic study. Laparotomy disclosed a 6 cm endometrioma of the left ovary, adhesions retracting the uterine fundus to the left, congenital absence of the right fallopian tube and a fibroma of the right round ligament. Additional endometrial implants on the bowel were fulgurated.

Comment: The numerous small adhesions affixing the left ovarian mass to the uterus are typical, though not diagnostic, of endometriosis.

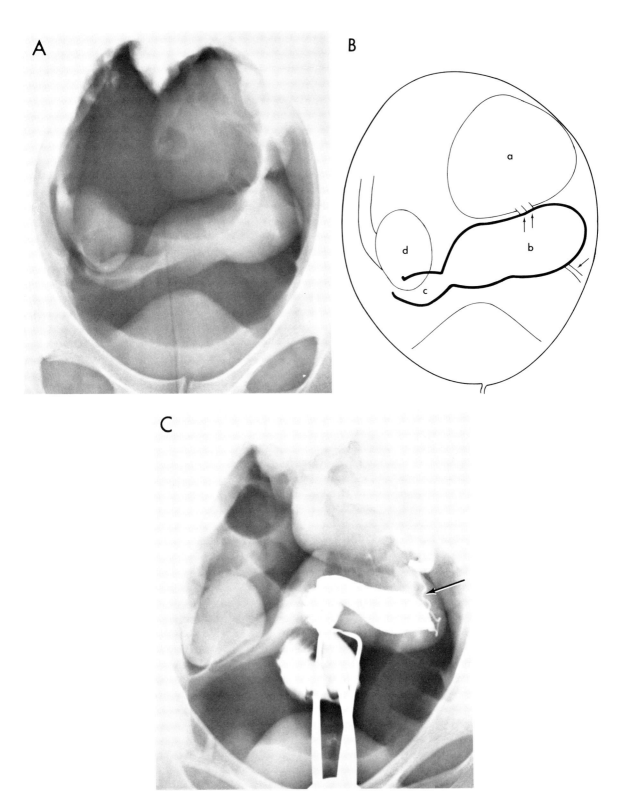

Figure 134 · Endometrioma / 307

Figure 135.—Missed tubal abortion simulating tubal neoplasm: uterosalpingograms.

A, anteroposterior view: Showing a large filling defect in the isthmus of the right fallopian tube.

B, right posterior oblique exposure: With contrast circumscribing the products of conception in a tubal pregnancy with missed abortion. The tube is obstructed beyond this site.

A gravida IV, para 1 patient, age 32, had her last menstrual period in November and experienced heavy vaginal bleeding two months later, in January. At that time, tissue was passed, presumably due to spontaneous abortion. A pregnancy test was positive the following April but another was negative in May. Intermittent bleeding occurred until June, when dilatation and curettage yielded negative results. Bleeding continued to occur until a second dilatation and curettage in September, when fractional scrapings from an "upper cavity" containing chorionic villi and decidua were obtained. Uterosalpingography was then done and demonstrated missed abortion in the right fallopian tube.

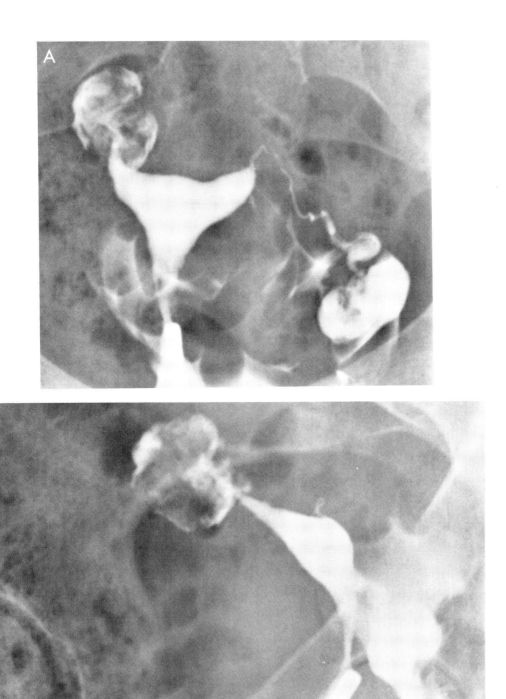

Figure 135 · Missed Tubal Abortion / 309

PART 4

Extrapelvic Tumor Extension and Recurrence

Techniques for Extrapelvic Tumor Extension and Recurrence

SUPPLEMENTARY METHODS for assessing reproductive tract tumor extension and recurrence outside the pelvis include lymphangiography and pelvic and caval venography. Neither method reliably opacifies the veins or lymphatics of the pelvis proper.

LYMPHANGIOGRAPHY

In the case of lymphangiography, catheterization of the dorsal foot lymphatics opacifies the external iliac and periaortic lymphatics but does not reliably delineate the internal iliac chain. Lymphangiography therefore plays no role in the diagnosis of primary tumors of the reproductive tract but is useful in detecting their extension or recurrence outside the pelvis. The technical aspects of lymphangiography including the procedure for performing catheterization and injection of the lymphatics are thoroughly discussed in the monograph by Fuchs, Davidson and Fischer.[1] It is essential to monitor the filling phase so that overfilling with resultant excessive embolization will not occur if high-grade obstruction is present. Films must be taken in the filling phase immediately after completion of the injection and during the storage phase 24 hours later. Anteroposterior and oblique exposures are customarily made.

The principal value of lymphangiography in assessing reproductive tract tumors is the demonstration of unsuspected nodal involvement which will influence treatment planning. It is important to remember that negative results will erroneously occur when metastases are too small to be identified (5 mm and less), are so large that the node is replaced by tumor or involve nodes which remain unopacified. Nodes may be skipped because of several anatomic irregularities: (1) occasionally major lymphatic channels are not linked directly with the primary regional nodes; (2) there may be direct anastomosis between afferent and efferent lymphatics; (3) some lymph node intermediate sinuses may be so large that they do not effectively act as a filter. False positive interpretations may result from fibrolipomatous involution of nodes (Fig. 143), granulomatous disease and hyperplastic inflam-

---

[1] Fuchs, W. A.; Davidson, J. W., and Fischer, H. W.: *Lymphography in Cancer* (New York: Springer-Verlag, 1969).

matory changes. Despite these limitations, a diagnostic error of only 15% had been reported by various experienced investigators when utilizing lymphangiography for staging carcinoma of the cervix. The accuracy of interpretation has been by no means uniform, however, ranging from 86–50% in various reports.[1, 2] The contribution of lymphangiography is seen in the fact that positive nodes are demonstrated by this means alone in 12–33% of stage I and II carcinomas of the cervix.

The accuracy of staging carcinoma of the uterine fundus, ovaries, vagina and vulva has also been significantly improved by lymphangiography in experienced hands.

Diagnosis of recurrent tumor is a vexing problem with the inherent limitations of bimanual pelvic examination as well as the difficulty of differentiating postoperative scar, postradiation effect, venous thrombosis and infection from neoplastic recurrence. Lymphangiography can be of great value in clarifying some such questions.

Venacavography and Pelvic Venography

Unfortunately there is at present no satisfactory way of opacifying, in the same procedure, both the pelvic veins and the inferior vena cava. Direct opacification of the pelvic veins has been accomplished via injection into the cervix or fundal myometrium, selective left ovarian vein catheterization and by reflux filling from iliac injection. The latter method is successful only when the internal iliac vein valves are congenitally absent, incompetent or so severely obstructed that contrast medium is forced into the pelvis. Injection into the uterus or cervix produces erratic symmetrical filling of the pelvic veins and is of dubious safety when a tumor involves the cervix or uterine fundus. These methods fail to opacify the external iliac veins and the combination of dilution and slow injection rate prevents opacification of the vena cava. The most commonly used practical venous assessment is limited to the external iliac veins and inferior vena cava and is well described by Ferris *et al.*[3]

Venacavography is generally performed via bilateral Seldinger catheterization of the femoral veins with subsequent injection of 40 cc of 60% Renografin (or its equivalent) using a Y connector. Catheters of PE 205 or 240 size are satisfactory and contrast is injected under relatively low

---

[1] Fuchs, W. A.; Davidson, J. W., and Fischer, H. W.: *Lymphography in Cancer* (New York: Springer-Verlag, 1969).

[2] Howatt, M.: Lymphangiography as an adjunct to gynecologic roentgenology, Seminars Roentgenol. 4:289, 1969.

[3] Ferris, E. J., *et al.*: *Venography of the Inferior Vena Cava and Its Branches* (Baltimore: Williams & Wilkins Company, 1969).

pressure (e.g., 150 psi). Anteroposterior, right posterior oblique and supine horizontal beam films are taken as required during suspended respiration but avoiding the Valsalva maneuver.[4]

Venacavography is a particularly useful supplement to lymphangiography because of the customary less complete filling of the right upper periaortic lymph nodes.[5] One must be cognizant of the location and appearance of the normal "washout" defects produced by the entrance of unopacified blood from tributaries to the vena cava (Fig. 139, *C*). Another source of confusion is the streaming effect of contrast. This is particularly obvious when the patient is horizontal and asymmetrical filling occurs due to successful catheterization of only one femoral vein or to venous obstruction on one side. Suggestions for overcoming some of these difficulties by upright venacavography[6] and by catheter modification[7] have been made.

[4] Mellins, H. Z., and Pischnotte, W. O.: Inferior Cavography and Pelvic Phlebography, in Schobinger, R. A., and Ruzicka, F. F. (eds.): *Vascular Roentgenology* (New York: Macmillan Company, 1964), pp. 538 ff.

[5] Baum, S., *et al.:* Lymphangiography, cavography and urography: Comparative accuracy in diagnosis of pelvic and abdominal metastasis, Radiology 81:207, 1963.

[6] Hayt, D. B.: Upright inferior venacavography, Radiology 86:865, 1966.

[7] Wendel, R. G.; Evans, A. T., and Wiot, I. F.: A new technique for inferior venacavography, J. Urol. 100:705, 1968.

Figure 136.—Recurrent carcinoma of the cervix with extension.

A, postinjection lymphangiogram, anteroposterior view: Showing obstructed lymph channels in the upper right iliac region (**a**) due to metastatic carcinoma of the cervix (proved by biopsy).

B, postinjection lymphangiogram, right posterior oblique exposure: Revealing the obstructed right upper iliac lymph channels (**a**).

C, 24 hour lymphangiogram, anteroposterior projection: Confirming obstruction of right common iliac nodes (**a**).

D, inferior venacavogram (injection via left iliac vein only), anteroposterior exposure: Demonstrating absence of inferior vena cava filling with extensive shunting into paravertebral venous collaterals due to metastatic carcinoma of the cervix in the region of the iliac confluence. The right ureter (**b**) is partially obstructed.

A gravida I, para 1 woman, age 41, developed postcoital bleeding which led to diagnosis of necrotic, infected stage I carcinoma of the cervix, for which radium and external megavoltage therapy was given. Two years later swelling of the right leg and obstruction of the right kidney developed. Findings on lymphangiography and venacavography led to additional radiation therapy. She died a year later.

Figure 136, courtesy of Dr. R. A. Castellino, Stanford University, Palo Alto, Calif.

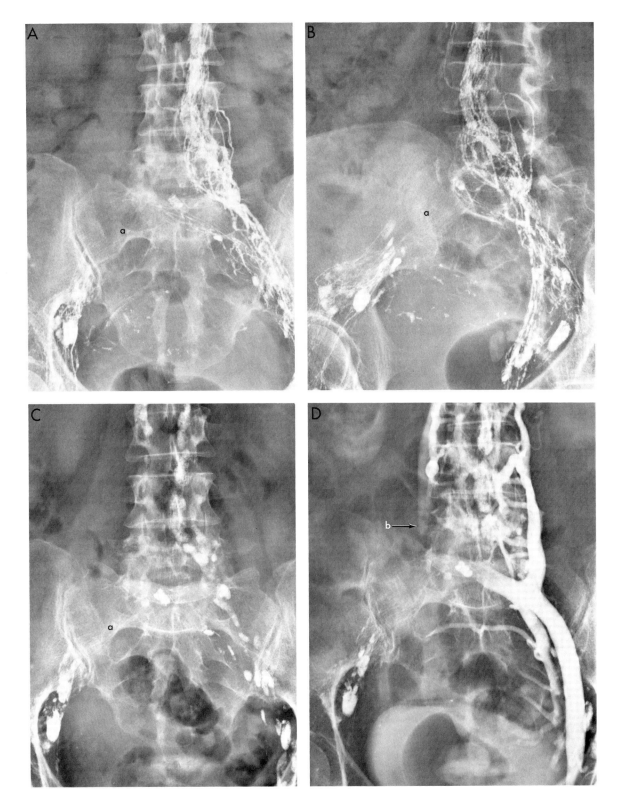

Figure 136 · Iliac Obstruction / 317

Figure 137.—Carcinoma of the cervix with extrapelvic extension.

A, 24 hour lymphangiogram, anteroposterior pelvic exposure: Showing pelvic collateral channels (**a**) filled due to iliac obstruction. Large lower right iliac nodes are seen with lack of filling of upper iliac nodes (**b**) due to metastatic tumor (proved by biopsy).

B, same lymphangiogram, abdominal exposure: Showing the right paraortic chain minimally filled, the left chain well filled.

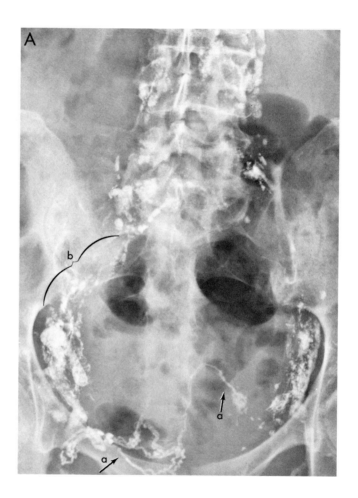

C, venacavogram, lateral projection: Demonstrating deformity and displacement of the vena cava at the second lumbar level (**arrow**) by enlarged metastatic right paraortic nodes which are not filled by lymphangiography (proved by biopsy).

A woman, age 53, with carcinoma of the cervix had lymphangiography and inferior venacavography for assistance in staging.

Comment: The complementary value of inferior venacavography and lymphangiography is well illustrated by the recognition of nonpalpable right iliac and paraortic metastases.

Figure 137, courtesy of Dr. R. A. Castellino, Stanford University, Palo Alto, Calif.

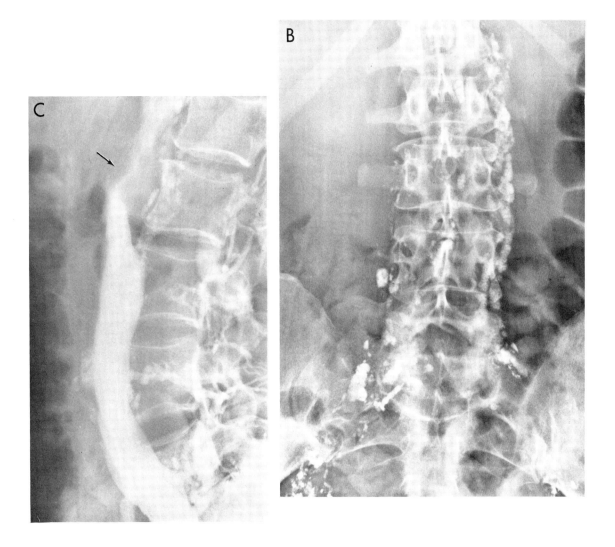

Figure 137 · Iliac Obstruction / 319

Figure 138.—External iliac vein obstruction secondary to carcinoma of the cervix.

A, venacavogram, anteroposterior projection: Showing no abnormality. Note that the catheter is advanced above the obstruction (**arrow**) of the left external iliac vein seen in **B,** thus giving misleading information.

B, pelvic venogram with catheter lower in the external iliac vein than in **A:** The obstruction due to recurrent carcinoma of the cervix is seen (**a**) and collateral channels are demonstrated (**b**).

C, pelvic venogram later in the series: Delineating the extent of the obstruction (between **a—a**) and shunt across the pelvis via the uterine veins (**c**).

A 47-year-old woman with stage Ib carcinoma of the cervix was given radiation therapy 16 months previously. In recent weeks progressive painless swelling of the left leg had resulted in brawny edema. Left lower extremity venography and lymphangiography showed no abnormality.

Figure 138, courtesy of Dr. R. A. Castellino, Stanford University, Palo Alto, Calif.

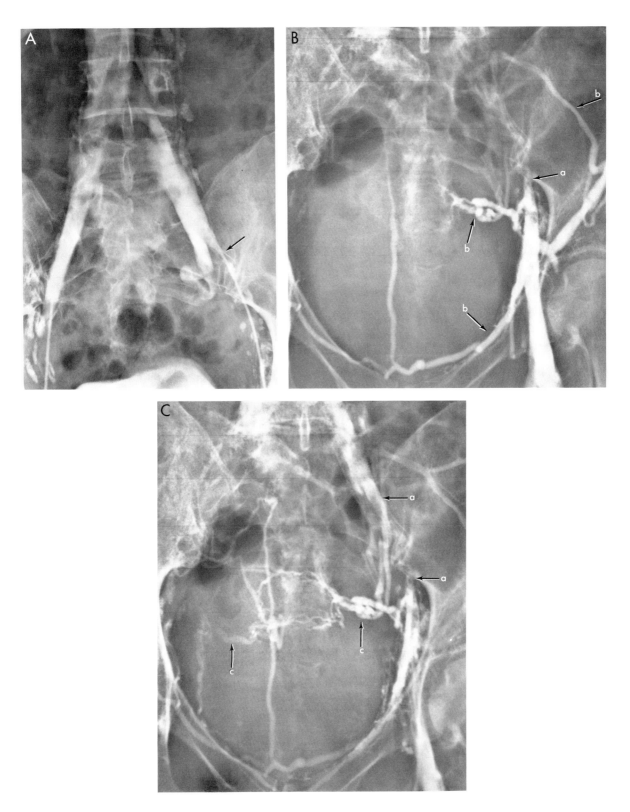

Figure 138 · Iliac Obstruction / 321

Figure 139.—Lymph node metastasis from ovarian carcinoma.

A, postinjection lymphangiogram, left posterior oblique projection: Revealing displacement of left iliac lymph channels (**arrows**).

B, 24 hour lymphangiogram, left posterior oblique projection: Delineating displaced nodes (**a**), node defects (**b**) and persistent lymph channels (**c**), indicating metastatic tumor in the left iliac and paraortic regions.

C, inferior venacavogram, anteroposterior view: Showing no abnormality. Normal renal vein washout defects are seen (**d**).

Until this 44-year-old woman developed flooding menstrual periods she had been entirely normal. Pelvic examination under anesthesia indicated a probable anterior uterine pedunculated fibroid. She continued to bleed and exploratory laparotomy was done. The "fibroid" proved to be a left ovarian, poorly differentiated serous cystadenocarcinoma. Hysterectomy and salpingo-oophorectomy were performed. There was no evidence of pelvic, abdominal or lymphatic metastasis. Classification of this tumor was changed from stage II (Rubin) to stage IV by the lymphangiographic findings. A 5300 rad pelvic and paraortic node dose was subsequently given.

Figure 139, courtesy of Dr. J. R. Eltringham, Stanford University, Palo Alto, Calif.

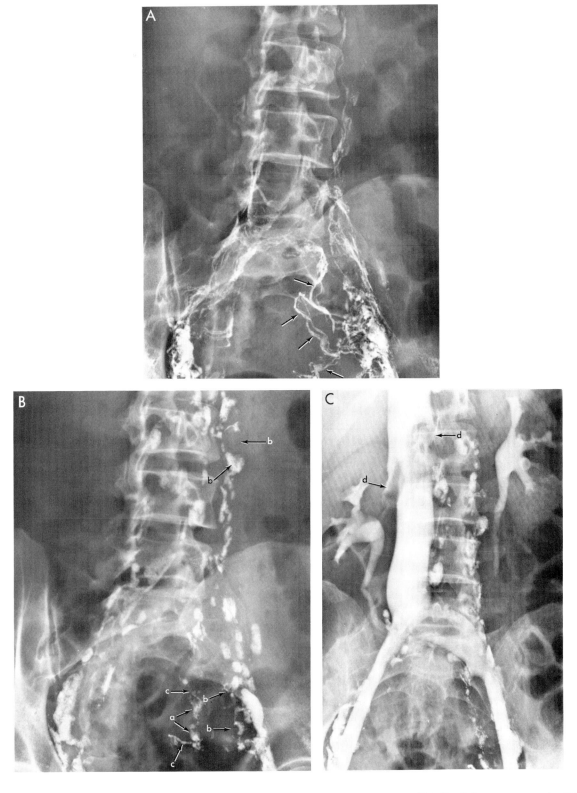

Figure 139 · Lymph Node Metastases / 323

Figure 140.—Lymph node metastases from ovarian carcinoma.

A, lymphangiogram, right posterior oblique projection: Demonstrating metastasis to the right upper iliac and paraortic nodes (**arrows**). The left side was not injected.

B, excretory urogram and lymphangiogram, anteroposterior exposure: Showing numerous lymph node metastases (**arrows**) and a large pelvic tumor compressing the urinary bladder and ureters.

C, inferior venacavogram, anteroposterior view: Delineating compression of the common iliac veins by the primary tumor and vena cava at the second lumbar level by metastatic nodes.

A woman, age 54, complained of abdominal discomfort and a mass in the lower abdomen. Excretory urography and barium enema disclosed a large pelvic mass and moderate right hydronephrosis. At exploratory laparotomy a well-differentiated serous papillary cystadenocarcinoma of the right ovary with left ovarian metastatic implants was found. There was no palpable evidence of metastatic disease in the abdominal viscera, omentum, liver or nodes. Hysterectomy and bilateral salpingo-oophorectomy were performed. The illustrated lymphangiograms assisted in identifying metastatic disease to the paraortic nodes. A 5460 rad dose was delivered to the pelvis in 39 days. The patient later had malignant pleural effusion.

Figure 140, courtesy of Dr. J. R. Eltringham, Stanford University, Palo Alto, Calif.

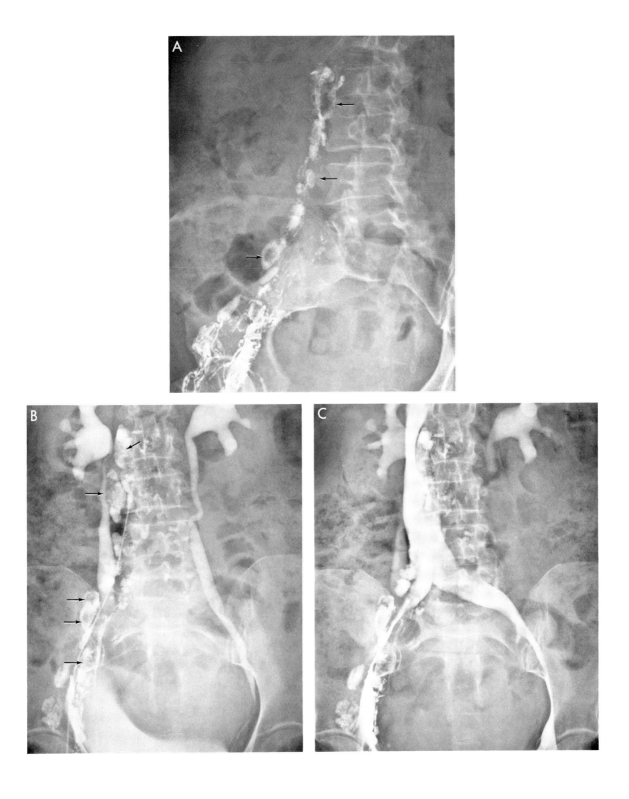

Figure 140 · Lymph Node Metastases / 325

Figure 141.—Metastasis to paraortic nodes from ovarian carcinoma.

A, 24 hour lymphangiogram, anteroposterior view: Showing nodal enlargement and persistent lymph channels extending to a point of partial obstruction in the left lower paraortic region (**arrow**).

B, lymphangiogram and inferior venacavogram, anteroposterior projection: The cavogram is normal. Negative excretory urogram.

Bilateral papillary serous cystadenocarcinoma of the ovaries was discovered in this patient in 1962, and hysterectomy and bilateral salpingo-oophorectomy were performed. No gross evidence of metastatic disease was

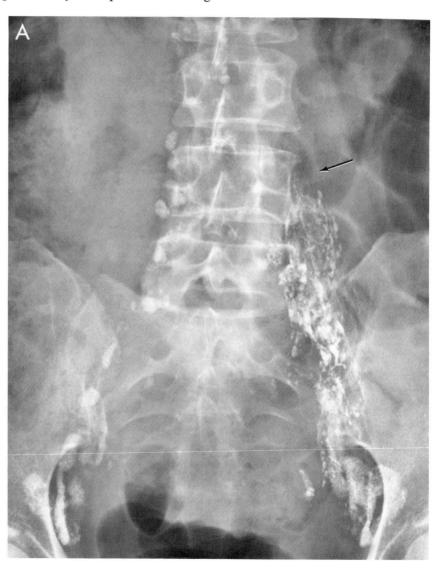

present at that time. Four years later, symptoms suggested recurrence and the illustrated radiographic studies were made. Surgical exploration confirmed the presence of involved nodes in the left paraortic region near the left renal hilus. With guidance from the lymphangiogram, a 5450 rad dose was administered to the retroperitoneal nodes. The patient died in 1968 after further recurrence of tumor in the pelvis.

Comment: Inferior venacavography is not reliable in the evaluation of left paraortic node disease, as shown in this case.

Figure 141, courtesy of Dr. J. R. Eltringham, Stanford University, Palo Alto, Calif.

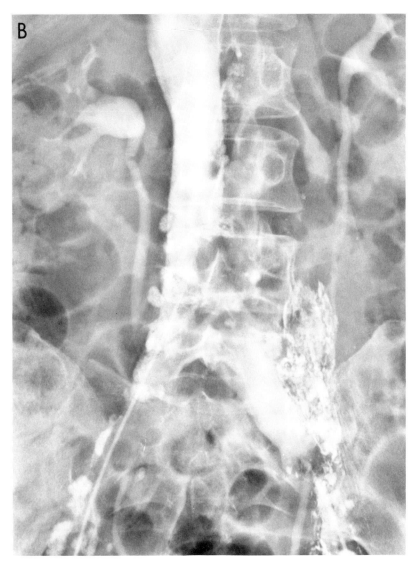

Figure 141 · Lymph Node Metastasis / 327

Figure 142.—Lymph node metastases from ovarian carcinoma.

A, postinjection lymphangiogram, anteroposterior view: Showing collateral lymph channels on the left (**a**) and early filling defects in several nodes (**arrows**).

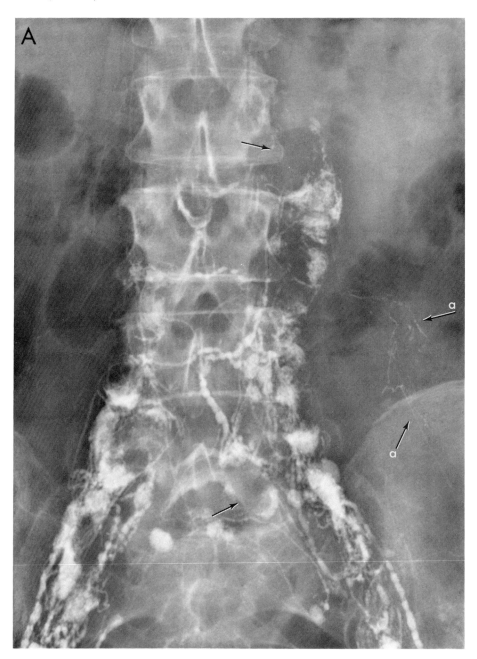

B, 24 hour lymphangiogram, anteroposterior projection: Revealing numerous metastatic node defects (**arrows**).

(*Continued* on page 330).

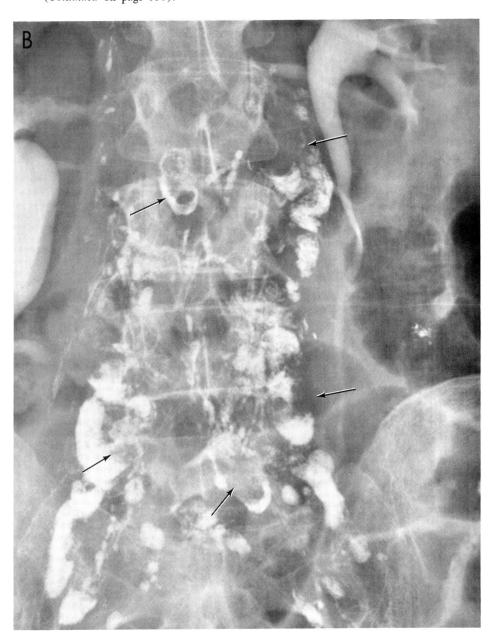

Figure 142 · Lymph Node Metastases / 329

Figure 142 (cont.).—Lymph node metastases from ovarian carcinoma.

C, inferior venacavogram, anteroposterior view: Disclosing extrinsic compression of the vena cava by metastatic nodes (**b**).

D, inferior venacavogram, right posterior oblique projection: Demonstrating metastatic node defects (**c**).

The patient, 62, had lower abdominal pressure leading to laparotomy and identification of a right ovarian, poorly differentiated cystadenocarcinoma. Following hysterectomy and salpingo-oophorectomy she was referred for radiation therapy. A stage III carcinoma of the ovary was thought to be present on pelvic examination. Lymphangiography showed extension beyond the pelvis, and 5500 rads was given to include the paraortic nodes. She died 19 months after completion of therapy.

Figure 142, courtesy of Dr. J. R. Eltringham, Stanford University, Palo Alto, Calif.

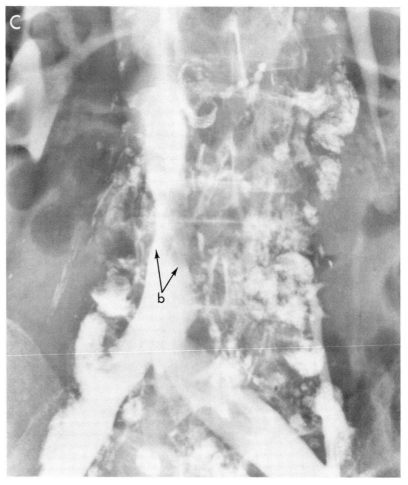

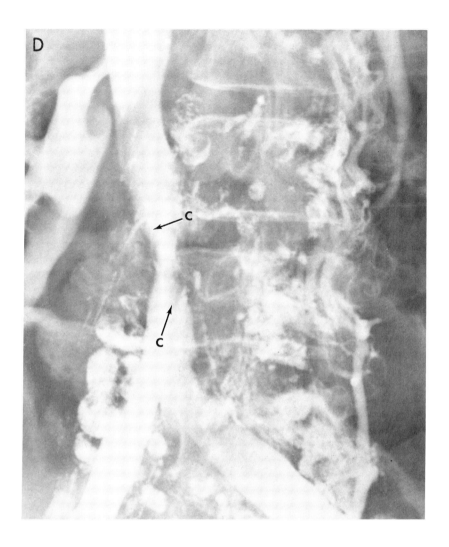

Figure 142 · Lymph Node Metastases / 331

Figure 143.—False positive lymphangiogram.

Twenty-four hour lymphangiogram, anteroposterior projection: Showing numerous central and eccentric filling defects in nodes of each iliac chain (**arrows**).

A 22-year-old woman had a routine preemployment physical examination and pelvic masses were palpated. Pelvic exploration was done and bilateral ovarian tumors were identified. The initial diagnosis was serous cystadenocarcinoma, and hysterectomy and bilateral salpingo-oophorectomy were done. After instillation of 60 mg of Thio-tepa in the peritoneal space, she was referred for radiation therapy. Some nodularity in the cul-de-sac and thickening of the left parametrial area placed the tumor in stage III category. The lymphangiogram was interpreted as showing probable metastasis.

Subsequent review of the pathology slides designated the tumors as serous cystadenomas rather than malignancy. On subsequent reexploration for clarification, no tumor was found. The defects noted on the lymphangiogram were produced by fibrolipomatous infiltration. The patient was well a year later.

Figure 143, courtesy of Dr. J. R. Eltringham, Stanford University, Palo Alto, Calif.

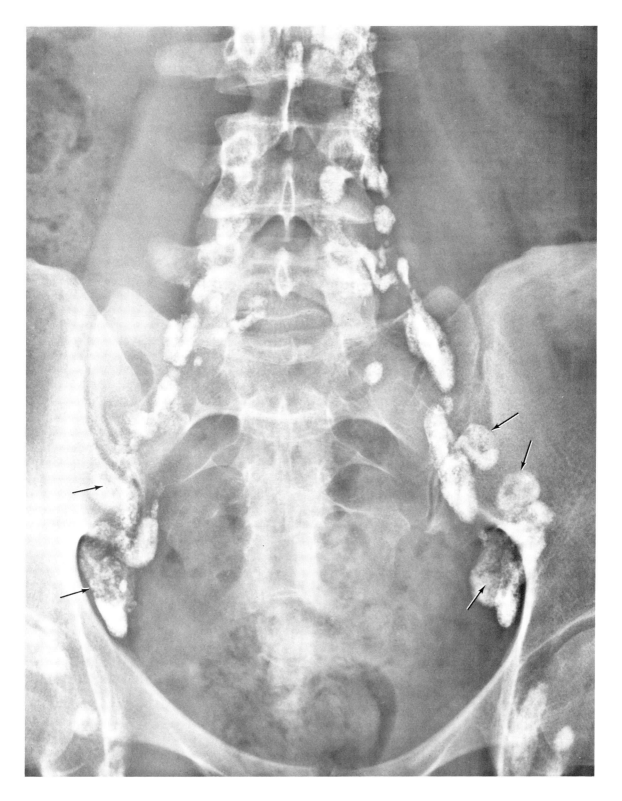

Figure 143 · False Positive Lymphangiogram / 333

Figure 144.—Lymph node metastasis from fallopian tube carcinoma.

A, 24 hour lymphangiogram, right posterior oblique view: Showing metastatic node defects at the second and fourth lumbar levels (**arrows**).

B, venacavogram (right iliac injection only), anteroposterior projection: Showing no abnormalities.

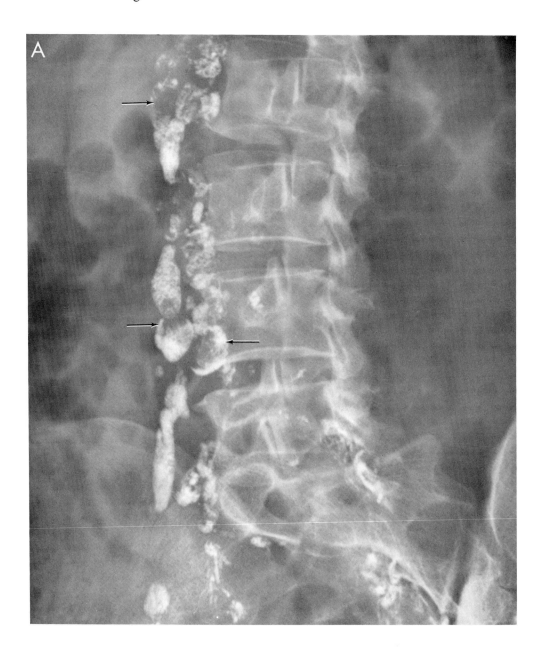

Five years after surgery and irradiation for adenocarcinoma of the left fallopian tube, the patient, 54, complained of pelvic fullness. Radiography before repeat surgery disclosed recurrent or new adenocarcinoma of the right adnexal structures. Palpably enlarged, firm, discrete nodes in the paraortic area and two nodules in the liver were found during surgery.

Figure 144, courtesy of Dr. J. R. Eltringham, Stanford University, Palo Alto, Calif.

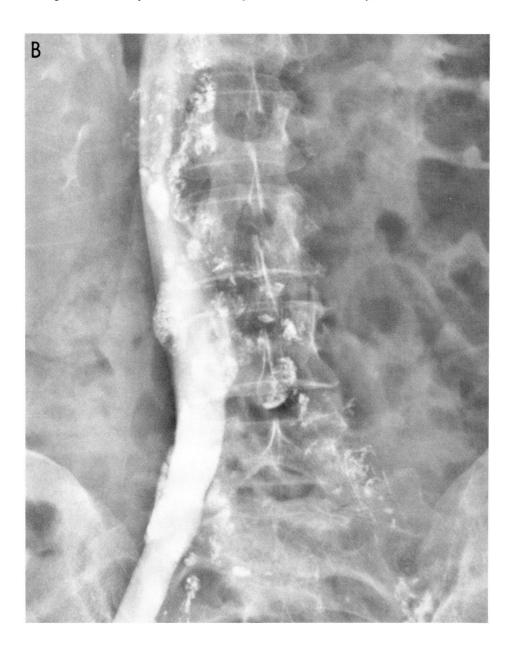

Figure 144 · Lymph Node Metastasis / 335

Figure 145.—Carcinoma of a fallopian tube with paraortic extension.

A, 24 hour lymphangiogram, anteroposterior view: Showing large foamy left iliac and paraortic nodes. Some nodes have metastatic defects (**a**), and lymph channels (**b**) bypassing obstructed nodes are seen.

B, 24 hour lymphangiogram, left posterior oblique projection: Demonstrating metastatic node defect (**a**) and lymph channels bypassing obstructed nodes (**b**).

C, inferior venacavogram anteroposterior view: Delineating extrinsic pressure defects on the left side of the vena cava (**c**) produced by paraortic lymph node metastasis (proved by biopsy).

D, venacavogram, right posterior oblique exposure: Showing scalloped deformity of the posterior left aspect of the vena cava (**c**) due to paraortic node metastasis.

A woman of 57 with history of carcinoma of the breast was found to have carcinoma of the left fallopian tube with extension to the sigmoid mesentery and right tube and slight ascites. Hysterectomy and bilateral salpingo-oophorectomy were done and she was referred for radiation therapy.

Figure 145, courtesy of Dr. R. A. Castellino, Stanford University, Palo Alto, Calif.

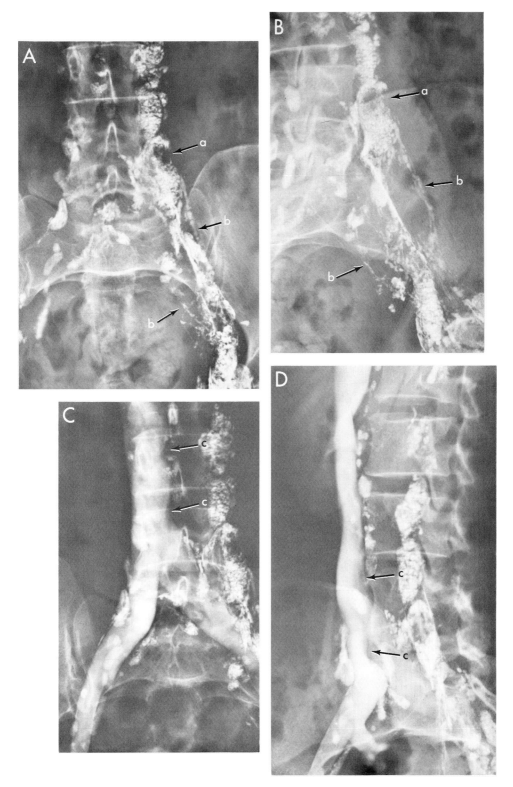

Figure 145 · Metastases to Paraortic Nodes / 337

Index

A

ADENOCARCINOMA, OVARIAN
with metastases, 266–67, 272–73
papillary, 240–41
bilateral, 272–73, 282–85
with calcification, 244–45
recurrent after therapy, 276–77
ADENOMYOSIS, UTERINE, 23
coexisting with endometriosis, 23, 170
AMNIOGRAPHY: technique, 118 f.
ANGIOGRAPHY, PELVIC, 7 ff.
in cervical carcinoma—extension and
recurrence, 96 ff.
normal arterial anatomy, 9, 18–19
technique, 8 f.
ARRHENOBLASTOMA, 180, 216–17
ARTERIES, PELVIC
with fibroids, 64–71
in hydatidiform mole, 119, 134–39
in invasive trophoblastic neoplasms,
122, 140–57
normal anatomy, 9, 18–19
ARTERIOGRAPHY, PELVIC, see Angiography
ASCITES: with cystadenocarcinoma, 236–
39, 254–55

B

BLADDER, URINARY
eccentric position causing pseudotumor,
172–73
normal
in pelvic pneumogram, 14–15, 40–41
in plain films, 3, 10–11
BRENNER TUMORS: bilateral, 222–23

C

CALCIFICATION(S)
in dermoid cysts, 182, 183, 186–87,
194–95
of fibroids, 25, 26–33, 36–41, 48–49
ovarian
in gonadoblastoma, 181, 224–25
in mucinous tumors, 179, 260–61
psammomatous, 179, 181, 224–25,
244–59
in serous adenoma, 179, 208–209,
244–59

CANCER; CARCINOMA
cervical—extension and recurrence
pelvic angiography in, 96 ff.
vascularity, 96
endometrial, 22 f., 76–79
in bicornuate uterus, 88
fungating, undetected by curettage,
89
pyometra with, 84–85
of fallopian tubes, 181
uterine
hysterography in, 74 ff.
—to follow response to therapy, 90–
93
pyometra complicating, 84–85
radium displacement, 92–93
undetected by curettage, 86–89
CERVIX
canal in uterosalpingogram, 16–17
carcinoma extension and recurrence
pelvic angiography in, 96 ff.
vascularity, 96
CHORIOADENOMA DESTRUENS (INVASIVE
MOLE)
see also Trophoblastic Tumors, invasive
diagnostic methods, 120 ff.
CHORIOCARCINOMA
see also Trophoblastic Tumors, invasive
diagnostic methods, 120 ff.
with metastases, 150–57
residual or recurrent after chemotherapy, 158–61
COLON, SIGMOID
diverticulitis, causing pseudotumor,
296–97
fluid-filled, causing pseudotumor, 291–
93
normal, in pelvic pneumogram, 14–15
CUL-DE-SAC OF DOUGLAS: in pelvic pneumogram, 14–15
CURETTAGE: in diagnosis of invasive trophoblastic neoplasms, 121
CYST(S)
ovarian
see also Cystadenoma
dermoid, 182 ff.
hydatid pedunculated, 212
nonneoplastic, 177 f.
of remaining ovary, 213

Cyst(s) *(cont.)*
    serous, 218–19
    —*see also* Cystadenoma
  parovarian, 181
    with bilateral ovarian fibromas, 228–29
Cystadenoma; Cystadenocarcinoma (Ovarian), 178 f., 204–09
  mucinous, 179, 204–207
  in postmenopausal patient, 264–65
  pseudomucinous, 204–205, 226–227
    with osseous metaplasia, 262–63
  serous, 179, 208–209, 236–41, 244–59
  in a child, 280–81
  with Meigs's syndrome, 268–69
  with metastases, 246–47, 250–53
  papillary growth in, 236–49
  psammomatous calcification, 208–209, 244–59
  20-year study, 258–59
Cystosarcoma Botryoides, 24
  in a male, 166–67
  of vagina, 162–65

D

Dermoid Cysts(s), 182 ff.
  calcification in, 182, 186–87, 194–95
  capsule sign, 182, 198–99
  fat (lipoid) content, 182, 194
  pedunculated, 188–89
  during pregnancy and after, 192–93
  with uterine fibroids, 190–91, 200–201
Diverticulitis: of sigmoid, causing pseudotumor, 296–97
Dysgerminoma, 180, 286–89

E

Endometrioma, 301–305
  with adhesions and fallopian anomaly, 306–307
Endometriosis, Ovarian, 178, 300–309
  with uterine adenomyosis, 170
Endometrium
  carcinoma, 22 f., 76–79
    in bicornuate uterus, 88
    fungating, 89
    pyometra with, 84–85
  hyperplasia, 22
  polyps, 22, 72–73
  sarcoma, 23
Enteritis: with intestinal loops causing pseudotumor, 290

F

Fallopian Tubes
  anomaly (absence), 306–307
  carcinoma, 181
  hydrosalpinx with tubal-ovarian mass, 294–95
  neoplasm simulated by missed tubal abortion, 308–309
  in pelvic pneumogram, 14–15
  pregnancy in, causing pseudotumor, 298
  tumors, 181
  in uterosalpingogram, 16–17
Fat Pad, Perivisceral: in plain films, 4
Fibroid(s), 25 ff.
  calcification of, 25, 26–33, 36–41, 48–49
  intraligamentous, 34–35, 50–51, 58–59
  with ovarian dermoid cysts, 190–91, 200–201
  in pregnancy, 62–63
  simulated by lithopedion, 60–61
  with uterine carcinoma, 80–81
  vascularity, 25, 64–71
Fibroma: bilateral ovarian, with parovarian cyst, 228–29
Fluid, Intraperitoneal: in plain films, 4

G

Gonadoblastoma, 180
  bilateral, with calcification, 224–25

H

HCG, *see* Human Chorionic Gonadotrophin Assay
Hemangiopericytoma (Myometrial), 23
Hematometra: bifid uterus with, 168–69
Human Chorionic Gonadotrophin Assay: in invasive trophoblastic neoplasms, 120
Hydatidiform Mole, 118 ff.
  amniography in, 118
  arteriographic features, 119, 134–39
  invasive (chorioadenoma destruens), 120 ff., 142–43
  pelvic arteriography in, 119
Hydrosalpinx: with tubal-ovarian mass, 294–95
Hysterography, *see* Hysterosalpingography
Hysterosalpingography
  with endometrial polyps, 72–73
  normal anatomy, 16–17
  technique, 6 f.
    to follow response to therapy, 90–93
    in uterine cancer, 74 ff.

I

INTERDIGITAL CREASE: in pelvic pneumogram, 14–15

K

KIDNEY: ectopic, causing pseudotumor, 299
KRUKENBERG TUMORS, 179

L

LEIOMYOMA, UTERINE, *see* Fibroid(s)
LIGAMENTS: in pelvic pneumogram, 14–15
LIPOMA: myometrial, 23
LITHOPEDION: simulating fibroid, 60–61
LUTEOMA OF PREGNANCY, 178, 210–11

M

MEIGS'S SYNDROME: serous cystadenocarcinoma with, 268–69
MESONEPHROMA: bilateral, 274–75
MUSCLE(S): iliopsoas, in plain film, 10–11
MYOMETRIUM—TUMORS
    adenomyosis, 23
    hemangiopericytoma, 23
    lipoma, 23
    myoma, *see* Fibroids

O

OVARY
    adenocarcinoma, 240–41, 244–45, 266–67
    carcinomatosis, 270–71
    cystadenoma and cystadenocarcinoma, 178 f., 204–09, 236–41, 244–69
    cystic enlargement, 44–45
    see also Dermoid Cyst(s)
    cysts
        corpus luteum, 177
        —hemorrhagic, 178, 214–15
        follicular, 177
        hydatid pedunculated, 212
        nonneoplastic, 177 f.
        parovarian, 181, 228–29
        of pregnancy, 178
        of remaining ovary, 213
        serous, 218–19
    endometriosis, 178, 300–309
        with uterine adenomyosis, 170
    normal
        in pelvic pneumogram, 14–15, 40–41
        in plain films, 3, 10–11
        in uterosalpingogram, 16–17

polycystic (Stein-Leventhal), 178, 220–21
reticulum cell sarcoma, 278–79
tumors of, 177 ff.
    characteristics, 177 ff.
    germ cell, 180
    gonadal stromal, 180 f.
    granulosa and theca cell, 180
    Krukenberg, 179

P

PELVIS
    normal anatomy (plain film), 10–11
    plain films—technique and interpretation, 3 f., 10–11
    pseudotumors, 290, 296–97, 299
PNEUMOGRAPHY, PELVIC
    normal anatomy, 14–15
    positioning for, 6, 12–13
    technique, 4 ff.
    pneumoperitoneum technique, 4 ff.
PNEUMOPERITONEUM TECHNIQUE FOR PELVIC PNEUMOGRAPHY, 4 ff.
POLYPS: endometrial, 22, 72–73
PREGNANCY
    in bicornuate uterus, 168–69
    corpus luteum of, simulating ovarian neoplasm, 230–31
    cysts of, 178, 210–11
    ectopic
        nonviable, simulating fibroid, 60–61
        tubal, causing pseudotumor, 298
    fibroids in, 62–63
    luteoma of, 178, 210–11
    twin—dermoid cyst during, 192–93
PSEUDOTUMORS
    ovarian-adnexal
        due to sigmoid loops, 291–93
        ectopic tubal pregnancy, 298
        endometrioma, 301–307
        hydrosalpinx with tubal-ovarian mass, 294–95
    pelvic
        due to bowel loops with enteritis, 290
        ectopic kidney, 299
        from sigmoid diverticulitis, 296–97
    uterine, 168–73
PYOMETRA: complicating uterine carcinoma, 84–85

R

RADIOGRAPHIC TECHNIQUES
    amniography, for trophoblastic tumors, 118
    hysterosalpingography, 6 f.

RADIOGRAPHIC TECHNIQUES *(cont.)*
    in uterine cancer, 74
   pelvic angiography, 8 f.
    for trophoblastic tumors, 119
   pelvic pneumography, 4 ff.
   plain films of pelvis, 3 f.
RADIUM MISPLACEMENT: in uterine cancer, 92–93
RECTUM: nomal, in pelvic pneumogram, 14–15

S

SALPINGITIS
   bilateral, 234–35
   unilateral, 232–33
SARCOMA: reticulum cell, of ovary, 278–79
SARCOMA BOTRYOIDES, 24, 162–67
SOFT TISSUES: pelvic, in plain film, 10–11
STEIN-LEVENTHAL SYNDROME, 178, 220–21

T

TERATOMA (OVARIAN), 180, 242–43
   benign cystic, *see* Dermoid Cyst(s)
   solid, 180, 242–43
TRANSVERSE VESICAL FOLD: in pelvic pneumogram, 14–15
TROPHOBLASTIC TUMORS, 118 ff.
   hydatidiform mole, 118 f.
   invasive trophoblastic neoplasms, 120 ff.
    angiographic features, 122
    diagnostic methods
    —curettage, 121
    —HCG assay, 120
    —pelvic arteriography, 121 f.
    metastasis survey, 122

U

URETER: in pelvic pneumogram, 14–15
UTEROSALPINGOGRAPHY, *see* Hysterosalpingography
UTEROVESICAL POUCH: in pelvic pneumogram, 14–15
UTERUS
   see also Endometrium *and* Myometrium
   bicornuate
    endometrial carcinoma in, 88
    pregnancy in, 168–69
   bifid, with hematometra, 168–69
   cancer; carcinoma
    hysterography in, 74 ff.
    —control studies to follow response to therapy, 90–93
    with myoma, 80–81
    pyometra with, 84–85
    radium misplacement, 92–93
    undetected by curettage, 86–89
   eccentric, with adnexal cicatrix (pseudotumor), 171
   in hysterosalpingogram, 16–17
   in pelvic pneumogram, 14–15
   in plain films, 3, 10–11
   pseudotumors, 168–73
   tumors and tumorlike conditions, 22 ff.
    endometrial
    —carcinoma, 22 f.
    —hyperplasia, 22
    —polyps, 22, 72–73
    —sarcoma, 23
    mixed mesodermal, 23, 94–95
    myometrial, 23

V

VAGINA: tumors of, 24